fit not healthy

How one woman's obsession to be the best nearly killed her

VANESSA ALFORD

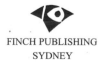

FINCH PUBLISHING
SYDNEY

Fit Not Healthy

First published in 2015 in Australia and New Zealand by Finch Publishing Pty Limited,
ABN 49 057 285 248, Suite 2207, 4 Daydream Street, Warriewood, NSW, 2102, Australia.

15   8 7 6 5 4 3 2 1

There is a National Library of Australia Cataloguing-in-Publication entry available at the
National Library.

Edited by Megan English
Editorial assistance by Catherine Page
Text typeset by Vicki McAuley
Cover design by Jo Hunt
Cover photograph courtesy of Vanessa Alford
Printed by 1010 Printing

Disclaimer
The events that have been written about in this book constitute my reality of what I went through.
Some facts may not be 100 per cent accurate, but they are as I saw them. If I have incorrectly
interpreted an event, consultation or discussion I apologise to anyone I may have offended.

The paper used to produce this book is a natural, recyclable product made from wood grown in
sustainable plantation forests. The manufacturing processes conform to Australian environmental
regulations.

Finch titles can be viewed and purchased at **www.finch.com.au**

Contents

	Foreword	v
	Prologue	1
1	2003 A pretty seaside town	4
2	2004 A healthy hobby	10
3	The Bangkok marathon	17
4	More than just fun	29
5	2005 Dangerously disciplined	39
6	Enter denial	47
7	The dream run	57
8	2006 Shattered	71
9	Warning signs	81
10	Breaking point	101
11	Consequences	107
12	Relapse!	126
13	Still searching for answers	141
14	2007 Despair	166
15	Desperate	180
16	2008 Adventure	187
17	Lessons not learnt	214
18	2010 Turning point	225
	Epilogue	239
	Acknowledgements	248

This book is dedicated with love to
Mum, Dad, Brent, Mia and Madison.

Foreword

Being fit is something many people aspire to. It is well known that regular physical activity has many health benefits. But can we have too much of a good thing? Can being too fit actually be detrimental to our health?

As a dietician, I often encourage people to increase the amount of physical activity they do along with making healthier food choices to assist in achieving health benefits. However, there is a growing trend of people taking the 'eat less, move more' message to excessive levels, and to a point where it no longer provides health benefits.

Restricting our food intake and increasing physical activity results in less energy or fewer kilojoules being available for bodily functions. If a very low amount of energy is available, the body is forced to rely on fat stores to function. In a situation where weight loss is warranted, this is desirable however, placing the body in energy deficit for a prolonged period of time is likely to have undesirable consequences. This is especially the case when entire food groups are removed, denying the body essential vitamins and minerals and forcing it to operate on a limited food supply. While following a restricted diet in the short term is likely to have minimal impact on one's health, depriving the body of vitamins and minerals over a prolonged period of time is likely to result in nutrient deficiency sickness. This is why following a balanced diet consisting of all the food groups is recommended.

Ensuring sufficient energy availability is particularly important for athletes who expend large amounts of energy through physical activity. Athletes are often conditioned to push their body to maximum levels and have the mental determination to adhere to follow extreme training regimes. However, our bodies also need rest and adequate fuel to function and perform at its optimum level and if insufficient kilojoules are consumed, this not only makes training counterproductive but may compromise the immune system and increase the risk of illness.

At times I have been faced with resistance when I remind athletes of the importance of refuelling their bodies adequately. Their desire to remain lean can often prove detrimental, especially when they are feeling fit, strong and invincible and fail to understand the importance of eating enough. This is particularly the case in sports where a low body weight is considered advantageous and there is pressure to maintain an 'ideal' body composition. I see this not only amongst elite athletes but also amongst other people whose desire to be lean results in them taking their exercise and diet to extreme, significantly compromising their health.

You are about to follow the sincere and heart-warming journey of a once healthy, moderate exerciser whose passion for running turned into a dangerous obsession. I congratulate Vanessa for writing and sharing an important and often silent aspect of an athlete's experience with food and training. Her raw honesty about her treacherous battle with her inner voice and revelations will inspire many and is a testament to her strength and integrity.

– *Anna Vassallo, Accredited practising dietician*

Prologue

Fit Not Healthy is my story from the age of twenty-two to thirty-two. But before I take you on my journey, I thought you should know about my childhood and adolescent years.

I was brought up by two loving parents – my French mother, who spent the first ten years of her life in Algeria, North Africa, before moving to Paris, and my English-born father, who has lived in Australia since he was ten years old. My parents met teaching in a school in London, married in Paris in 1973 and then moved to Australia. They spent another couple of years teaching in London where I was born in 1979. My younger brother was born in Melbourne four years later.

I can confidently say that my brother and I had the most fulfilling childhood: we were given a rich education, travelled extensively (including regular trips to France) and enjoyed the experience of a lifetime backpacking through East and North Africa and road trips through the US, New Zealand, Spain, Italy and Switzerland, all before the age of thirteen. I had visited over twenty-five countries by the time I turned eighteen, with many of our travels to developing countries. It made me realise how fortunate we are to live in Australia, compared to the devastating conditions in which some people live.

For as long as I can remember, sport has been my passion. I have always loved watching it and enjoyed participating even more. I began gymnastics at the age of six, and at seven I joined a netball team. At the age of ten I discovered tennis, which soon became my greatest devotion. I have vivid memories of changing outfits in the back of the car while my parents drove me from gymnastics to netball every Saturday. Sunday was taken up with tennis.

I was born to compete. My gymnastics team won the Victorian championships in the under-ten age group and my netball team won the state championships two years in a row in my last two years of primary school. My love for tennis and netball continued throughout high school, where I explored a number of other sports: diving, athletics, basketball and badminton.

I have always thrived on setting myself physical challenges. At the age of seven I climbed Ayers Rock (now known as Uluru) with my family and I vividly remember using every ounce of energy to complete the climb in the shortest possible time. At the age of twelve I often spent afternoons cycling laps of our neighbourhood, which included an enormously steep incline; once or twice was never enough – I'd set myself the challenge of doing so ten to fifteen times, until my legs were burning.

Running was never my favourite pastime. In fact, I really didn't enjoy it and found plenty of excuses to avoid going for a run; but I did make an effort to run five kilometres a few times per week to maintain my fitness for tennis and netball. It was always an effort to get out the door but the adrenaline rush at the end made it all worth it. I am naturally muscular and at 160 cm, I am definitely not in the tall category, but my regular training kept me at a healthy weight throughout high school. There were girls leaner and taller than me, but I was content with my body.

After graduating from high school in 1997, I began a bachelor of physiotherapy the following year. The regular socialising and drinking that came with being a university student added a few kilograms to my physique but this didn't bother me; I was having fun. During my first year of university, I was introduced to pole vaulting. My 'not quite voluptuous but slightly curvy' physique was not ideal for the sport and I never excelled, but I loved the training involved: weight training, gymnastics and sprint training. I continued to run five or six kilometres three times a week. Occasionally I ran eight or ten, which gave me a tremendous sense of self-satisfaction and achievement. But if I missed a session, it didn't matter. Overall, during my four years at university, I led a balanced lifestyle, finding time for regular training sessions in between (some) studying and (a lot of) socialising. Life was great.

When I asked friends to describe me using just one word, they mentioned driven, focused, motivated, courageous, strong-minded, ambitious and perfectionist. I have always been a high achiever, motivated by a strong desire to excel in all areas. For me, failure has never been an option. Praise from others is not what drives me, however, it is the sense of achievement, fulfilment, self worth and pride I feel. I aspire to new challenges. In fact, the greater the challenge put before me, the more driven I become. I thrive on going far and beyond what is expected of me and of eclipsing even my own expectations. If I want something, I don't wait for it to come my way, I use my initiative to go after it. And I will endeavour to do whatever it takes to make it happen – at all costs.

These are all desirable traits, one would think. But as you are about to see, in excess, they can culminate in a dangerous obsession that leads to self-destruction.

1

2003 A pretty seaside town

In December 2002 I graduated as a physiotherapist from the University of Melbourne. Two months later I moved to Townsville, where I started my first full-time job. Why Townsville? I don't really know. I wanted to live somewhere different to where I had lived the last twenty-one years of my life, so when a physiotherapy position became vacant at a sports medicine clinic in Townsville, I applied. After two telephone interviews, I was offered the position. This left me with an important decision to make: do I leave Melbourne, my friends and family and move to a remote town in the north of Queensland where I don't know anyone, where everything is foreign and where the population equates to that of a few Melbourne suburbs? Or do I stay in Melbourne, where family and friends are abundant, surroundings are familiar and the nightlife is vibrant?

I compiled a list of pros and cons for each option. For me, the only downside of moving to Townsville was being away from family and friends. The more thought I gave it, the longer my list of pros became: I would be living by the beach, winters would be warm, it would be a fantastic experience to live and work elsewhere, I would make new friends, the cost of living would be less and the position I had been offered was a great opportunity. If things didn't work out, I could always move back home – Melbourne would always be there.

My decision was made easier when a good friend from school,

who I had known for nearly ten years, was also offered a job in Townsville. So in January 2003, Jemma and I packed our bags and moved to the remote seaside town in North Queensland. Although I was a little apprehensive at moving to a new town, having company made the process a lot less daunting, and I was excited at the prospect of beginning a new chapter in my life.

I have only great memories of my time in Townsville. The locals were friendly and welcoming and I made lifelong friends. Jemma and I found a compact two-bedroom apartment metres from the beach, with a modest balcony overlooking a sparkling swimming pool. The town delivered such a relaxed ambiance that I felt like I was on an extended holiday and work was just a way to fill my weekdays. Weekends were spent jet skiing, sailing and taking leisurely drives to nearby towns.

Townsville is also where I began to develop a love for running and although I was unaware of it at the time, it was also when a healthy hobby began to transform into an obsession. It was where my desire to be fast and lean and push my body hard intensified; and little did I know at the time that it was to lead me on a harrowing, seemingly endless journey.

Before moving to Townsville, I was running a few times a week to keep fit, but it never took priority over partying, socialising or sleeping in. I would never think of setting my alarm for an early morning run. So when, during my first week in Townsville, a colleague assured me I would start running early in the morning to beat the heat, I instantly replied, 'No way. I would never get out of bed for a run.'

During my days as a university student I was renowned for staying in bed until early Sunday afternoon after being out late on a Saturday night. Large amounts of alcohol were often consumed and the festivities often ended a little messy in the early hours of Sunday morning. Although no longer at university, I still looked forward to eventful Saturday nights to help me unwind from the working week.

Two weeks after moving to Townsville there was a five-kilometre fun run held called 'The dash for cash'. The winner collected three hundred dollars. The start line was located conveniently in a large park across the road from our apartment, fitted with a children's playground, sandpit and swings. I decided to enter. I wasn't so sure about the early morning start, but I knew I would feel great after the run. I had agreed to meet a colleague at the start line at 6 am, but when I stumbled home from a night out at 3 am, my head spinning, I knew there was no way I would make it to the start line. My alarm clock sounded at 5.30 am, but I hit the snooze button and went straight back to sleep.

I couldn't have imagined that this would be the last time partying and sleeping took priority over running. I don't know what triggered the change, but over the weeks that followed I began to enjoy running more and more. For a few weeks I continued to party on Saturday night and managed to drag myself out of bed for an early morning run only a few hours after returning home. I felt seedy and hung over for the first few kilometres, but sweating out the remnants of alcohol that remained in my blood made me feel a lot better. There were a couple of Saturday nights where I stayed home and a had a good night's sleep instead, and no alcohol made for a more enjoyable run the following morning.

Over the next few months I found my early morning runs more and more invigorating and it didn't take long to realise that avoiding a big night out made my weekends much more enjoyable. Within a year of living by the beach in warm, sunny Townsville, I had become a different person. I still enjoyed socialising, but never until the early hours of the morning, and my days of sleeping in until 1 pm were a distant memory.

I set my alarm for 6 am every morning during the week and by 6.10 I was out the door, running my usual eight kilometres along the beach, watching the sunrise illuminate the pretty seaside town. There was no better way to start the day; breathing in the freshness and perfume of the oxygenated air provided me both peace and exhilaration at the same time. I thrived on the adrenaline that pumped around my body during and after a run. Nothing else could give me the same level of satisfaction. In fact, the more challenging the run, the greater the feeling of accomplishment I experienced.

I was home by 7 am, which gave me sufficient time to consume a hearty breakfast before cycling fifteen kilometres to work. I had ridden to university and work the past four years and I had never considered it exercise, but rather a way to commute. My eight-kilometre runs gradually became ten kilometres; and on weekends, I ran twelve kilometres. Following my longer runs on the weekends I rewarded myself with a big stack of pancakes. There was no guilt after having expended so much energy. My mind was clear and I was ready for the day ahead.

After a couple of months of regular running, I began to notice changes in my body. I considered myself a little chubby the past couple of years and would have happily lost five kilograms to reach my ideal weight, but I didn't care enough to do anything about it. I was happy and enjoying life so I didn't see any reason to change.

Growing up I had always eaten well. My parents enforced good habits from an early age but I have always enjoyed donuts, chocolate and ice cream as treats and never held back. But as my running mileage increased, my diet became healthier ... and healthier. I began consuming more fruit and vegetables and eliminating foods high in fat and sugar. The changes weren't intentional; they just happened. After a couple of months if I felt like sugary foods I didn't even consider donuts or chocolate; fruit and yoghurt were now my 'sweet fix'.

Within six months, I had shed a layer of fat from my body and by the end of the year, I had effortlessly lost six kilograms and dropped a clothing size. People noticed and the compliments flowed. My new, lean physique and improved fitness were gratifying. I felt a zest for life that I hadn't previously known. I couldn't imagine my life without running and felt something missing if I didn't begin the day with a run. I gradually increased the distance of each run. What's another two kilometres? I asked myself. And another two? Just one more. Before long my twelve-kilometre weekend runs had become twenty. It was effortless.

I had discovered a love for running that I previously didn't know existed so when a friend from work suggested I enter the Townsville Marathon in August that year, I was easily convinced. I was running the distance of nearly a half marathon every weekend anyway, so I had no doubt that I could run forty-two kilometres with a few months of training.

I began by adding two kilometres to each Sunday run, then one Sunday in July, I completed thirty-eight kilometres. Although a little nervous, I felt prepared and confident as I stood at the start line of my first marathon three weeks later. I had been advised by a colleague who had experience running marathons not to go out too hard. 'Just find your rhythm and go at your own pace,' was his advice. I did exactly that and had a great experience, finishing in a respectable time of three hours thirty-five minutes. I felt fit and strong. I felt invincible.

Following my first marathon I decided I never wanted to return to my previous weight and began taking an interest in the number of kilojoules I consumed each day. I didn't know the exact kilojoule content of every food so it was only an estimate, but I soon began researching the kilojoule content of different foods. I kept track of the kilojoules I consumed at breakfast, lunch and dinner. I still allowed myself occasional treats, but they became less frequent. I ran every day, partly because I loved it and craved the adrenaline rush, but also because it meant I could enjoy treats without guilt while still maintaining my new, slender physique.

Rewarding yourself with an edible treat after a tough workout is nothing unusual and it keeps people motivated, so I didn't consider this train of thought unusual. I was as healthy as I had ever been. What I didn't realise was that this mindset and my desire to control my kilojoule intake would consume my thoughts tirelessly for years.

2

2004 A healthy hobby

I had met my boyfriend, Brent, some years earlier, when I was 15, as we lined up on opposite sides of the net at a local tennis club in the eastern suburbs of Melbourne. We were playing mixed doubles in a junior tennis competition and, as I prepared to return serve, I couldn't help thinking how attractive my opponent was. His six-foot-three stature was impressive, and I found his piercing, ocean-blue eyes, wavy brown hair lightened by the sun and breathtaking smile extremely appealing. I made a point to remember his name and was pleasantly surprised a few months later when I met his older brother while working at the Australian Open. We both worked at 'Fan fest', where anyone could come and join in the various tennis activities, including testing the speed of your serve. It was also where players appeared to sign autographs. I became good friends with Brent's brother and we kept in touch.

Brent and I crossed paths at parties and at tennis tournaments and, as we became friends, I became attracted to more than just his appearance. His laid-back attitude and charisma complemented his Tom Cruise-like looks and I found myself wanting to spend more time with him. Our friendship developed but, despite his name being scrawled all over my Year 11 diary and hints from Brent that he was interested in more than just a platonic friendship, this didn't eventuate. 'I'll call you,' he would often say to me when we met. But he never did.

Six years on, my schooling and university degree completed,

we were still in touch but had only met up once or twice a year as he had spent the past two years coaching tennis in New York. Having seen very little of him, I thought I was well and truly over my 'high school crush' – but when Brent sent a group email to his friends suggesting we visit him at the five-star resort he was living and working at on one of the most exquisite beaches in Thailand, I jumped at the opportunity. Not only to see Brent, but who could knock back a free stay at an exclusive resort in Thailand?

Three weeks later, I landed in Phuket, and within two days our platonic relationship had developed into much more. While I was very happy, I did wonder if the relationship was just 'convenient' for Brent and had happened only because all his friends were thousands of miles back home. But my doubts were erased after I had returned home and he told me on the phone how much he missed me and asked me to come back to Thailand. I spent every penny I had to fly back to Thailand for another three weeks. As we were preparing to say goodbye once again we both realised how strong our feelings had become for each other.

Brent and I maintained a long-distance relationship for most of my year in Townsville, although he did manage to visit me for two weeks in March and September in between his six-month positions as a tennis coach in Thailand and New York. We spent a total of four weeks together that year. People thought it was ludicrous that we remained a couple when we were physically apart for so long, but I didn't care what anyone else thought. There was no-one else I wanted to be with and the times we did spend together were worth the long months apart. But after nearly twelve months, with no end in sight to our long-distance relationship, I began to question how long we could continue with thousands of miles between us.

It was just before Christmas, eleven months after I had moved to Townsville, when I brought up the issue during our nightly phone call.

'Come to Thailand,' was Brent's immediate response. 'Come and live with me here. I miss you too much. You can find a job teaching English. That way we will be together.'

This was not as far-flung and out-of-the-blue an idea as it seemed. Brent knew that teaching English in a developing country was something I had always wanted to do. On top of this I would be finally with my boyfriend who was halfway across the world, and living in a five-star resort in Thailand! I would be able to run along the beach every morning, eat pad thai and enjoy delicious banana and mango shakes every day. I didn't have to think about it for too long and a little over two months later, in February 2004, I headed to Thailand. I was sad to leave Townsville and the great friends I had made, but it was time for a new adventure.

Two weeks before my departure, Brent called to tell me he was entering the Bangkok Marathon with some of his colleagues. He asked if I wanted to join him. Of course! I was ready to conquer another marathon and to run it faster than my last one. 'Register me,' I blurted out without a second thought. The challenge had been set before me and I couldn't wait to go for my next run.

I was concerned, however, about Brent running his first marathon as he hadn't run further than eight kilometres in the past few years. His job as a tennis coach meant that he had basic fitness, but anyone who has run a marathon is well aware that forty-two kilometres is not just five times more demanding than running eight kilometres. It is about one hundred times more strenuous on the body. It is a test of mental and physical endurance that requires you to switch off your body's pain receptors and test your limits. Pounding the pavement continuously for three or four hours and depleting your fuel tank in the process requires training. A lot of it. Your body needs to prepare for torn muscle fibres and depleted glycogen stores, dipping into fat stores and potentially breaking down protein to fuel the last few kilometres. I was worried he might not finish the race.

'I'll be fine,' he said when I voiced my concern. 'I have two months to train. That's over eight weeks. I'll increase the distance of my long run by three or four kilometres every week so by race day, I'll have run thirty-six kilometres.'

His response was a true reflection of Brent's casual and positive attitude towards everything in life. Just another thing I loved about him. I didn't want to burst his bubble and loved the idea of running a marathon together so quietly agreed it was possible …

I arrived in Thailand at the beginning of February where a surreal lifestyle welcomed me. We had four swimming pools, three tennis courts and the ocean at our doorstep. I was overcome with excitement, not only about the incredible lifestyle I was going to have but the exhilaration I experienced as I ran into Brent's arms for the first time in five months.

'I've missed you so much,' he cried, holding me tight, refusing to let go. 'I'm so glad you're here with me.'

'Me too,' was all I could manage as I kissed him, while trying to hold back tears of joy. Finally we were together. And this time it would be for more than just two weeks.

In 2004 I was at a healthy weight. I was aware of the kilojoules I consumed and expended but I was not fixated on them. I was running regularly because it was easy, enjoyable, and provided me with more relaxation and stress release than sitting on the couch watching television. I couldn't wait to run along the beach each morning, to inhale the fresh air and feel the salty ocean spray against my skin. The adrenaline would flood my body and a feeling of euphoria (supposedly similar to the elation experienced from cannabis) would sweep over me. I couldn't get enough.

Running also provided me with a simple way of keeping my weight low. This was important because the resort's main restaurant put on an amazing buffet breakfast every morning of bacon and eggs, croissants, cakes, donuts, fruit, yogurt, pancakes, waffles ... The list was endless and my favourite pastime meant I could indulge in delicious delicacies without worrying about piling on the kilos. I expended kilojoules running, so I had earned the right to consume them.

The heat and humidity in Phuket is similar to Townsville, so I wasn't concerned that I only had six weeks to acclimatise before the marathon, but the furthest I had run since the Townsville marathon six months earlier was twenty-five kilometres. I knew I needed more long runs under my belt and I wanted to stand on the start line confident that I could not only finish the race, but that I could run it faster than my first marathon. I would not accept a slower time. I knew that if I had any doubt in my mind about whether I could complete the distance, I would begin the race mentally defeated. I had to believe I could do it.

I had planned to resume training the day after I arrived in Phuket, but I woke that morning with a throbbing headache, feeling nauseous and fatigued. I had been recording each run I completed since the marathon in Townsville and realised I had not had a day off running for ten days. I had even managed to squeeze in a run a few hours before flying to Thailand. My body was telling me it needed rest, so I listened and spent the next few days relaxing by the pool and swimming in the ocean. I enjoyed watching the children splashing around in the pool, squealing with delight while their parents, basking in the sun nearby, watched on. I limited the treats I ate during those few days, aware that I was burning very few kilojoules. I missed my daily runs and felt lazy, but I knew it was for the best.

Five days of relaxation later, I felt refreshed and rejuvenated. Over the next week, in between teaching five hours of English each day at an International language centre in Phuket town, I completed three five-kilometre runs and a ten-kilometre run. While losing weight hadn't been my initial motivation for running, I loved how it was stripping off layers of body fat. Brent's colleagues commented on how fit I looked compared to the previous year and how fluent my strides appeared. The compliments on my athletic, ripped physique enhanced my self-esteem and sense of self-worth. There was no way I wanted to return to my previous, curvy self.

The following Sunday I ran twenty four kilometres. I then increased my long run each week until I was comfortably running thirty-six kilometres. I covered the same twelve-kilometre loop three times and left my drinks at the start so I could rehydrate every twelve kilometres. I preferred to run on my own so I could run when I wanted, the route I wanted and most importantly, at my own pace. Since running the Townsville marathon I had been advised by a few other runners to begin incorporating interval sessions into my training program to improve my speed. I had given it some thought, but I didn't feel any need to put myself through the pain of interval sessions. I had never been a sprinter and the idea of running flat out around a running track made my hair stand on end. My love of long-distance running was growing by the day and although I was hoping to run the Bangkok Marathon faster than my previous one, I was content with how things were going and I didn't want to start putting too much pressure on myself. But one week before the marathon, I surprised myself by completing thirty-six kilometres in under three hours – less than five minutes per kilometre. I looked at my watch in disbelief. I felt fast, fluent and light and couldn't wait for the challenge of running faster than ever.

3

The Bangkok marathon

Two nights before the Bangkok marathon Brent and I were invited by friends to a carbo-loading party of pasta, pasta and more pasta. The theory behind carbo-loading is that you load up on carbohydrates to fuel your body with as much glycogen as possible before the race. It's rather like filling your car with petrol before a long road trip. We went to the party, but I was not there for the food. As ridiculous (and possibly rude) as it may have seemed, I brought my own rice and vegetables.

'You didn't need to bring anything. We have everything covered,' the host of the party said as he opened the door and gestured us inside.

With a sense of guilt, I explained to him that I had eaten the same meal the two nights before every long run and I didn't want this one to be any different. Call it superstition, but I didn't want to fill my stomach with a big bowl of starchy pasta that it was not used to digesting. He raised his eyebrows as his eyes widened, obviously a little surprised, but his pleasant smile indicated he wasn't offended.

My other reason for not wanting to carbo-load was that the week leading up to a marathon, you reduce your training load to prepare for the race. You want to line up at the start feeling well rested, without fatigue or muscle soreness. This is called tapering. Instead of running eighty kilometres that week, you might only run twenty to thirty kilometres and by maintaining your diet, you load your body with the extra kilojoules usually expended in training. Consuming additional carbohydrates on top of this would essentially be excessively overloading your body. The more glycogen the body stores, the more water that is stored, resulting in an increase in overall body weight. I didn't want to begin the race feeling heavy, so while others indulged in large bowls of pasta, I was content with my bowl of rice and vegetables.

Brent happily accepted the pasta on offer and as I watched him down mouthfuls of spaghetti I couldn't help but think about his less-than-ideal preparation for his first marathon. Since deciding to enter the race two months earlier he had gradually increased his weekend runs to thirty-two kilometres. In addition, he completed a couple of ten-kilometre runs each week, after being on the tennis court for five hours each day. I was still worried he wouldn't finish the race but it was too late to say anything now and to complement Brent's optimistic attitude towards everything in life, I wanted to remain positive.

The following afternoon we flew from Phuket to Bangkok with two other couples, both a few years our senior and all but one person running their first marathon. Our flight was delayed and we landed in Bangkok at 4.30 pm, exactly twelve hours before the start of the race. It was a two-hour drive to our hotel and we had arranged to pick up our race kits at 6.30 pm. I wasn't happy about arriving late when the race began at 4.30 am the next day. I would have preferred to arrive earlier in the day or the day before even, to have time to orientate ourselves, find a restaurant that served vegetables and rice (not difficult in Thailand) and have time left over to relax.

Our race preparation could not have been worse. The van that was supposed to pick us up from the airport was nowhere to be seen and it took over an hour of frantic phone calls before our driver eventually picked us up. Worse, he didn't speak English and as the van weaved in and out of the horrendous Bangkok traffic, the blare of horns deafening, we had no idea if we were heading in the right direction. At around 7 pm I was relieved to see a sign indicating that we were heading towards our destination but an hour later, having turned in circles and with our driver looking increasingly worried, it was obvious we were lost.

With the race beginning in a little over nine and a half hours, I was beginning to get anxious. It was approaching my dinnertime, too. I had never eaten dinner after 8 pm the night before a long run and I didn't want this to be any different. My stomach was aware of exactly how much time it had to digest dinner before the run. I began to feel hungry and I could feel my muscles stiffening.

I looked at Brent. He was glancing at our friend beside him who was on the phone to one of the race organisers. We had been told they would wait for us to collect our race kits, but we had no doubt they had packed up and gone home. No-one spoke. Nothing needed to be said. The poor lighting made it difficult to read street signs. I was on the edge of my seat and could feel my muscles become tighter and tighter, totally unable to relax. What a nightmare, I thought, wondering if we would make it to the race at all.

I had given up on getting a decent amount of sleep. At this rate, we would be in bed after midnight, less than three hours before our 3 am wake-up call. After several phone calls and numerous stops to refer to a map, illuminated with a torch that he found in the glove box, our driver found his way to our hotel. I was furious, but restrained from displaying any hostility. As all Thai people are, he was very friendly and obviously didn't understand the urgency of the situation.

We climbed out of the van, exhausted and hungry, and were greeted by the event organisers and hotel staff. Thankfully they had stayed to wait for us. They handed us our race kits – our bib, timing chip and a few snacks – and the key to our rooms, and told us dinner was ready for us in the hotel restaurant. Aware of the time and not in any mood to make conversation, Brent and I wearily made our way to our room.

I was becoming increasingly anxious by the minute. It was now close to 9 pm. I wondered if I should go straight to bed so I could at least get some sleep before the race, and save my body the task of having to digest my dinner in time. However, as I hadn't eaten for six hours I followed Brent to the restaurant and joined the others, who were tucking into their bowls of rice and vegetables. Someone must have known I was coming, I thought. There wasn't the quantity or variety I was used to, but it was more than I had expected. We ate in silence and when we were finished, we went back to our rooms. Brent and I unpacked our running gear, placed it neatly on a chair, brushed our teeth, kissed each other good night and crawled into bed, too tired to say much. I looked at my watch, which said 9.45 pm. Our wake-up call was a little over five hours away.

I was woken by three loud knocks on the door and a voice calling, 'Wake up. The race is in ninety minutes.' No way, I thought. Surely the night can't be over already. The night wasn't over for most, in fact, as it was completely dark outside. I felt like I had just crawled into bed. It was times like this that I wondered why I put myself through such torture. Why would I voluntarily wake up at 3 am to run forty-two kilometres? For the love of it? The challenge? As crazy as it sounds, yes. For the adrenaline rush, the jubilation and the enormous pride and sense of fulfilment that envelops your body as you cross the finish line. It is why people keep coming back for more, despite the agonising pain during the last few kilometres. It makes running marathons addictive. I had been given a taste of it in Townsville and couldn't wait for more.

Come on, I urged my body. Wake up. Getting up for an early run had never been so difficult. I felt physically exhausted, mentally drained and my muscles were stiff. I could still taste last night's dinner and didn't have a good feeling about the race. The knocking became louder. 'Yes, yes, we're awake,' I called, speaking for myself and Brent, who was still lying in bed, tucked under the sheets. Just looking at him made me want to close my eyes and roll back to sleep.

I crawled out of bed, my eyes half closed, and stumbled to the bathroom. I threw cold water on my face then put on my running gear. I checked that Brent was awake and told him I would meet him in the van. I preferred to be alone before the race so I could prepare mentally, visualise myself gliding through the air and finishing the race strong.

By 3.30 am, we were ready to go. Just as the driver was starting up the van – the same driver as the night before, which immediately sent my heart racing – Brent realised he had forgotten something. 'Wait,' he cried with hint of urgency. 'I've forgotten my PowerBar.'

'Quick, we're already running late,' I snapped unintentionally as he jumped out of the van and ran back to our room.

He returned minutes later, PowerBar in his hand. A little out of breath, he climbed into the van. He sat beside me, placed his hand on my leg and smiled with a 'don't stress, we'll get there on time' look on his face. I was not totally convinced. However, we were finally on our way.

I wanted to arrive at least thirty minutes before the start to have ample time to warm up and go to the toilet, but the hotel wasn't as close to the start as I had anticipated and we arrived with only twenty minutes to spare. The entire lead-up to the race could not have been more stressful. It was a recipe for disaster. Brent clearly had a different attitude, looking as relaxed as ever during the trip, and chatting to the others on the bus. I stayed quiet, trying to control my nerves and focus on the race I wanted to run. I sat and stared out the window, avoiding any conversation and sending out clear signals to everyone not to talk to me. As soon as we arrived, we both joined the long queue for the portable toilets.

My biggest fear before any race is that I won't be able to go to the toilet. (It is so important to get it all out beforehand to reduce the chance of having to go during the race.) After waiting in line for ten minutes, it was my turn, but I couldn't go. Our late dinner had totally confused my body. I was so worried that I would need to go during the race, but with only five minutes until the start, I tried to erase this from my mind.

'Everyone please line up at the start line,' a voice said over the loudspeaker, first in Thai and then in English.

As I lined up next to Brent I glanced around at the other runners. I had been told there were participants from England, Germany, the US, Canada and France, but as foreigners, we were clearly the minority. I nervously jumped up and down on the spot, stretching the same muscles over and over. I knew my nerves would disappear as soon as the race started. Brent appeared far more relaxed; if he was feeling nervous, he certainly wasn't showing it.

'Ten, nine, eight, seven, six, five, four, three, two, one … Go!'

We were off. There was no turning back and no point worrying about my far-from-ideal lead-up to the race or what my bowels might decide. For the next three and half hours, hopefully less, it was me against the clock. It was dark; the path was poorly lit by the occasional street lamp. I focused on the person in front of me to prevent veering off track.

Although Brent and I planned to run at a similar pace, he knew I preferred to run my own race. I would be happy to run alongside him if it turned out that way, but I didn't want to commit to staying together.

The one piece of advice I will give anyone running their first marathon is to run your own race. This means running at your own pace: the speed you have trained for and feel comfortable at. A common mistake people make at the beginning of a marathon is to go out too fast. They try to keep up with those around them and without realising it, they run the first kilometre faster than they have ever run before. Forty-two kilometres is a long way and this overzealousness can come back to haunt them in the later stages of the race when absolute fatigue and exhaustion take over the body and glycogen stores deplete, causing them to 'hit the wall'. This has forced runners to finish marathons walking, staggering or even crawling.

There is also a significant risk of dehydration and electrolyte depletion during long-distance running that can result in dizziness, nausea, impaired concentration and in severe cases, hallucinations and collapse. In the later stages of a marathon, it is hard to know how close you are to reaching this point, which is why it is so important to have covered the actual distance you plan to run in training.

At the ten-kilometre mark, I was feeling great and Brent and I were still running together. 'Feeling good?' I asked.

'Okay,' he replied. I sensed a little unease in his voice, which contrasted with his usual 'I'll be fine' attitude. I didn't respond – nothing I said would make him feel more comfortable and I knew now wasn't the right time to talk about his far from adequate preparation. 'You?'

'Great!' I replied enthusiastically. He looked at me and smiled, a look of encouragement on his face in amongst the pain I knew he was feeling.

'You can do it,' he said.

'You too,' I replied, doing my best to sound reassuring. 'I know you can.'

A turnaround at the fifteen-kilometre mark revealed how many runners were ahead. At that stage I was placed tenth out of the female runners and I noticed a group of four women quite far in front. They had gone out fast and I estimated they were on track for a sub three-hour time. Wow, they must be elite runners, I thought. I wasn't in this race to win so I concentrated on myself, my pace and staying in the zone.

At 6 am we were welcomed by the rising sun, which provided us with more visibility than three metres ahead. We could now appreciate the beautiful scenery as we ran past traditional Thai temples and through rice fields. There were water stations every five kilometres where children played the drums, danced and sang. Men and women cheered. There were times when I wished I had my camera, but I was not there to play tourist. I was there to run forty-two kilometres and improve on my previous time. To my competitive self, any slower was not an option.

At the twenty-kilometre mark, I was still feeling strong and ready to increase the pace. Brent had dropped back, aware of his limits. He was not aiming for a particular time; he just wanted to finish the race. I had noticed a pack of men about fifty metres ahead so I asked Brent again how he was feeling and when he replied 'Okay' I put my foot on the accelerator to catch them. I was still feeling comfortable at the thirty-kilometre mark and another turnaround point at thirty-two kilometres affirmed I had closed the gap considerably on the four women. Two kilometres later, they were no more than two hundred metres in front. Don't get too excited, I thought. Run your own race.

Over the next three kilometres I bridged the gap further and at the thirty-six-kilometre mark, I flew past them. Their raised shoulders and laboured breath were clear indications that they were feeling the effects of having gone out too fast and that fatigue was setting in. Despite intense pain in both my calf muscles, I increased my pace with less than five kilometres to go. At the forty-kilometre mark the pain was extreme. I began to feel a little weary, but I could taste the finish line so I accelerated once more. A motorbike appeared alongside me at forty kilometres, a photographer perched on the back.

'Can we follow you to the finish line?' he yelled out.

'Sure,' I yelled back.

There are brief moments in life when you get a taste of what it feels like to be a celebrity, of people wanting a piece of you and watching your every move. This was one of those moments. I tried to enjoy it, despite the pain taking over my entire body. Come on, I told myself. You're nearly there. I felt a strain in my right calf as I ran past the forty-one-kilometre mark but I did my best to ignore it. The crowd had cheered me on during the entire race and I used all their energy to propel me to the finish line. The camera lens was still in my face and I tried to manage a smile as I turned the last corner, running down the home straight.

With a sudden surge of adrenaline I sprinted across the finish line in a personal best time of 3:20. I had run the last two kilometres faster than any other. I was handed a token. Second place. I couldn't believe it. Only the number one Thai runner who had crossed the line six minutes earlier had beaten me. I was ecstatic.

After receiving congratulatory slaps on the back and drinking over two litres of fluids, I waited at the finish line for Brent. I saw him turn the corner and head for the finish line just under four hours after we started the race. An amazing accomplishment by anyone's standards. I could tell he was hurting, but his mental toughness had got him over the finish line before his colleagues. He ran straight into my arms.

'What a run,' was all he could say.

That's all that was needed to be said. No words were required to sense each other's pride both for ourselves and for each other.

One hour later I was back at the twenty-one-kilometre mark having photos taken in front of traditional Thai temples, their horn-like projections representing the mystical Thai culture and adding to this already memorable experience. The photographer on the motorbike was from a German running magazine and asked if he could write a story on me. A professional photographer will take hundreds of photos before he is content and this one was no exception. I was asked to run past several temples numerous times, stopping between each shot so he could review the photos. My legs felt more painful than during the race as I had cooled down and my muscles were beginning to tighten up.

After what felt like hours, the photographer said he was satisfied with the photos and we drove back to the finish line for the presentation. I proudly walked on stage as my name was called to accept my trophy and cheque for second place. I couldn't wipe the smile off my face as I posed for the myriad of cameras.

As I soaked in the attention from what felt like hundreds of pairs of eyes and the perpetual clicking of cameras, I became suddenly distracted from the lenses in front of me. From the corner of my eye, I saw Brent collapse. As he fell into the arms of two people by his side, I leaped off the stage and ran to where he lay. He looked pale, all colour drawn from his face, beads of sweat sprinkled across his forehead. Thankfully, his eyes were open and he was responsive. The race doctors were by his side and assessing him in seconds. It wasn't long before they inserted a needle into his arm to administer a drip.

'He'll need to lie here until the drip has finished draining into his blood,' one of the doctors informed us.

'How long will that take?' I asked.

I had already held the rest of our team up by having to wait around for the presentation and I knew they were eager to return to our hotel – and I couldn't wait to jump in the pool to help alleviate the pain in my legs.

'About thirty minutes,' the doctor replied.

He explained that Brent had suffered severe dehydration and electrolyte depletion as a result of excessive sweating and inadequate rehydration. The solution draining into his arm contained the fluid and electrolytes to replenish his body. Thirty minutes later, the colour having returned to Brent's face, we scrambled into our van and were driven back to our hotel. Fully clothed, we all jumped straight into the pool.

Six hours later, after another ninety-minute bus trip, a two-hour flight and what felt like endless hours waiting around, we landed at Phuket airport. As I walked off the plane, it felt as if every muscle fibre in my legs had been torn. My calf muscles were as tight as a rubber band on full stretch and I wondered if they would ever return to their original length. I knew it was going to be a painful few days, but well worth it.

I rang my parents from the airport to share my excitement. Mum and Dad have always supported my brother and I in everything we do and they are the type of parents who feel like they can never do enough for us. They supported me in running marathons although deep down I knew they weren't entirely pleased with the idea, due to the risks involved in pushing the body so far. My mum answered the phone.

'How did you go?' she asked nervously.

'I came second!' I explained, my bubble of excitement growing by the second.

'That's wonderful, well done,' she replied. 'We are both very proud of you.' I knew she meant this but I could hear in her voice the relief that I had survived my second marathon. I hadn't hit the wall, I hadn't collapsed and I hadn't been taken off on a stretcher. I also detected slight concern as she knew this result would only motivate me to compete in more marathons. She knew I would want to run faster. To train harder. To push my body further. This, I knew she was not so thrilled about.

4

More than just fun

Two months after the Bangkok marathon and after teaching English for three months it was time for Brent and I to relinquish our dream life and return home to Melbourne – but not for long. Two weeks after arriving in Melbourne, Brent flew to New York for another summer of coaching. I knew I would struggle to live through Melbourne's cold, wet winter after having lived in warm, humid climates for over a year so I returned to Queensland to work – five weeks on the Gold Coast followed by two months in Townsville. After having lived together for a few months, being apart wasn't easy for either of us. The first few days in Queensland I was miserable and wanted nothing but to pack up and fly to New York to be with him. The days were long, the nights lonely. Brent felt the same way, as he was also living alone and working long hours, on the tennis court every day from dawn until dusk.

'All day, while I'm hitting balls I just think of us being together again,' he said to me during one of our nightly phone calls. 'It's what gets me through each day.' Brent would get up at 5 am, which was 9 pm in Queensland, to call me. I was thankful we could speak every day but not being able to see him or feel his touch was almost too much to bear. During this time apart, our feelings for each other grew stronger and we counted down the days until we would see each other again.

Living alone made me even more focused on my running. It intensified my passion and fuelled my hunger for more. I also had more time to think about my diet and maintaining my marathon-runner's body. Brent had never said anything about the amount I was running leading up to the Bangkok marathon, but I wondered if he thought I was overdoing it. I was almost certain that even if he did think I was doing too much, he would choose to remain quiet to keep the peace. And I was too scared to ask him, fearing what I might hear. Regardless of what he thought, in Queensland I was living alone so I could run as much as l wanted and no one would know. No-one except myself. Every morning I woke up at 5 am and headed straight out the door for a ten-kilometre run. I was home by 6 am for breakfast and then I rode to work for a 7 am start. The mornings were crisp, but by the end of my run I could feel the rays of the sun warming my skin. On weekends I had more time so I ran fourteen to sixteen kilometres in preparation for the Gold Coast Half-marathon, which I completed the week before leaving for Townsville. I finished in a personal best time of 1 hour and twenty-nine minutes. I felt in control of my body for the entire race. Running had never felt so good.

The following week, eighteen months since arriving in Townsville for the first time and exactly one year after completing my first marathon, I returned to the quiet seaside town to work at the same sports medicine clinic. I planned to work there for two months before flying to New York to meet Brent. It was great to see my colleagues, who all commented on my slim appearance.

'You look even thinner than when you left Townsville last year,' one of them said as soon as she saw me.

'You obviously haven't stopped running,' another said.

You wouldn't dare tell someone they look fat or have put on weight, but there is never any hesitation in saying someone looks thin. Initially, I took it as a compliment and it gave me a sense of satisfaction, but after a while, the tone in people's voices changed and they might as well have said, 'Have you eaten lately?' In hindsight, the tone in their voices didn't change, but my interpretation did. I took it personally. Deep down I knew I should be fuelling my body with more, but I didn't want to concede control over what went into my mouth, and my performance so far had not suffered – if anything, I felt I was running better than ever. So each time I just responded with a smile. Having done well in Bangkok and now looking like a marathon runner, I felt compelled to embrace this new identity. My runner's body reflected who I was and I wasn't about to relinquish it. At the same time, my hunger for competition and my desire to be the best had escalated.

My stay in Townsville coincided with the Townsville marathon and I was ready to give the local race another go. This time I wasn't there to just reach the finish line. I was there to eclipse my previous best time and finish faster than the other runners. I hadn't changed my training much over the past year – I still ran ten to twelve kilometres most days of the week, did a long run on the weekends and had no desire to do any interval training – but I was running faster than the previous year. The race was six weeks into my stay, which gave me ample time to acclimatise to the heat and humidity of the tropics.

Running in Townsville did not compare to running on the Gold Coast. In Townsville, you sweat profusely, so the risk of dehydration is far greater. Adequately hydrating during the race could mean the difference between finishing and collapsing before the end. I practised drinking fluids during my training sessions, especially during my long runs. I would leave a drink in my letterbox as I had done in Phuket and run the same loop three or four times, drinking fluids each time I completed a loop. I also ate one or two PowerGels during my training runs to replenish my glycogen stores.

As I warmed up for the race, it occurred to me how different things were compared to the year before. I was not searching for other runners who looked like they would be slower than me in fear of finishing last. This time I was looking for women who would pose a threat to a podium finish. The previous year's winner was there to defend her title – it was going to take a miracle to beat her – and I kept telling myself to ignore her and to stay in the zone. Just run your own race, I reminded myself.

I politely made my way to the front – another stark contrast from the year before when I had deliberately stayed at the back of the pack of runners – retied my shoelaces and did some final stretches before the countdown began. 'Three, two, one … Go.'

For forty-two kilometres I was in the zone, ignoring everyone around me, enjoying the sounds of nature, the smell of the trees, the freshness of the air, focusing on my breathing and just running my own race. As I had done in my previous two marathons, I finished strongly, totally in control of my body. I crossed the finish line in 3:07 and in second place, pumping my fists in the air, knowing I had smashed my previous personal-best time by thirteen minutes. I had given it my all and doubted I could ever run any faster.

However it wasn't long before I had created a new goal: to break the elusive three-hour barrier.

A week after the Townsville marathon I flew to New York to meet Brent, who was finishing his summer of tennis coaching. We had planned this earlier, which helped us to get through the months we spent apart. We both saved enough cash during this time to travel for several months. After two weeks in New York, we spent one week in Jamaica then travelled around Central America for four months. Brent returned home for a family Christmas while I spent six weeks on my own in India. I have always revelled in travelling on my own – Egypt, Norway, Sweden, Denmark, Laos and Cambodia and India in particular has always intrigued me.

Travelling solo can be lonely at times but also incredibly fulfilling; a liberating and thrilling experience that gives you the freedom of not having to consult anyone. It pushes you out of your comfort zone and forces you to talk with strangers. However, having travelled with Brent for four months, the first couple of weeks by myself were miserable. I missed having a companion, someone to share the experiences with, to laugh and cry with. I missed Brent's positive attitude – the way he never let anything get to him during the more challenging times, especially the arduous thirty-hour bus trips on rough terrain squashed in amongst other passengers, the freezing temperatures, the endless days surviving on chicken and rice. The way he would put an arm around me and reassure me everything would be okay when I felt down. During this time I decided to write a journal, as a way of expressing my feelings and sharing my experiences. A journal would be willing to listen and not judge me. This journal, which ended up going far and beyond my trip to India, would become a blessing in the years that followed.

14 December 2004

Despite its mystery and beauty, travelling through India as a single white female has proven to be no holiday. The persistent

*hassling is exhausting and the poverty-stricken streets are
emotionally draining. There are beggars on every corner and
they gaze at me with sunken eyes, their empty hands reaching
out for coins. I put a few coins into a pair of hands today but
the man was obviously not satisfied with the amount I gave
him because he threw them down and began yelling at me.
I couldn't understand what he was saying but it was frightening
so I continued walking, occasionally looking back over my
shoulder to make sure he wasn't following. I am so lonely —
too many hours alone. Too much time to think about Brent
and what he's doing back home. He's away with his mates
right now, probably having the time of his life. I wonder if he's
thinking about me at all. Is he even slightly worried that his
girlfriend is travelling around India alone? Does he miss me?
I hope so.*

During the six weeks, the days reached as high as forty degrees and
the nights were not much cooler. I endured painfully long bus and
train trips in atrocious conditions. My most gruelling train trip was
scheduled to take thirty-three hours, but unforeseen delays meant
it took forty hours to reach our destination. I had heard many
horror stories from travellers who had found themselves in hospital
with food poisoning only to have their condition deteriorate due
to the horrendous hospital conditions, so I refrained from eating
anything but rice and fruit. I left India having avoided Delhi
belly but I also lost weight – six kilograms to be exact. My weight
plummeted to a dangerous forty-three kilograms.

I knew I looked unhealthy (in retrospect some would have
described me as a walking skeleton), but a part of me was not

shocked by my new look. Actually, I was beginning to like it and couldn't wait to put my skinny jeans on when I returned home. I also liked the thought of needing to put on weight. But during my trip to India, a voice had begun to emerge in my head that would do everything to stop me from doing so. Initially it was there only at night, ensuring I didn't indulge in anything sweet after dinner, but each passing day it became a stronger, more frequent presence until it accompanied me everywhere I went.

My next stop was Paris, where I was reunited with my family for Christmas. My mother is French and she and my father, brother, grandparents, aunties, uncles and cousins were spending Christmas together. They couldn't and didn't hide their shock at my appearance. 'You're all skin and bones,' my mother gasped, grasping at her short black hair, her eyes wide with horror, as I walked out of the bathroom with a towel draped around me. My once-muscular arms and broad shoulders were waif-like, my shoulder bones protruding. I ignored the comments and brushed off any concern my parents had about my eating habits. Even my father, who usually let my mother do all the worrying, made the occasional remark about my weight.

'I've just spent six weeks in India. I'm fine. Stop worrying,' I repeated several times a day. 'I'll put the weight back on in no time.'

I knew I could get back to a healthy weight if I really wanted to – it was Christmas and every day I was tempted with delicious French delicacies such as croissants, pain au chocolat and crepes – but the voice became stronger, its authority more absolute. It ordered me to count every kilojoule and warned that putting on a few kilograms may lead to a snowball effect. It gave me permission to eat only after exercising. Looking at my hip and shoulder bones protruding and the sunken look on my face, I tried to ignore the voice, certain that the words were ludicrous. But I felt a sense of satisfaction as I pulled on my skinny jeans with ease.

Despite obeying the voice's commands and staying away from the French delicacies, I ate normal meals while I was in Paris, as I didn't want any of my family to become aware of my obsession with what I was eating. I returned to Melbourne after two wonderful weeks in Paris, having added three kilograms to my slender frame. But when I clocked in at forty-six kilograms, I was determined not to put on any more weight. I was staying at my parents' place and my mother made daily comments about my weight. 'You look so thin!' she would say. 'I'm worried about you.'

Although I knew her concerns were only because she loved me, I didn't want to hear it; my defensive response was the same every time, that I had just returned from India.

Brent was also unable to hide his shock at my frail appearance after I returned to Melbourne. He hesitated when I stepped forward to hug and kiss him. 'Look at you, you have lost so much weight!' he exclaimed. 'Your pants are baggy.' He had a genuine look of concern on his face but I failed to recognise this, instead hearing only a nagging voice telling me to eat more.

'I know, but I'm fine,' I replied abruptly. 'It's because I've just been to India.' After that, he rarely mentioned anything about my weight. And if he did, I shut him down with the same harsh response.

I knew deep down that I was too thin, but as I felt great within myself, I was not about to concede more kilos. I wanted to make sure that I continued to look like a marathon runner. Extreme measures in India had taken me below my ideal weight so I knew

I would have to continue a similar disordered way of eating to maintain it. I researched the kilojoule content of every single food and completely eliminated certain nutrients from my diet – first went the bad fats (trans and saturated fats), which were already scarce, then the good fats (monounsaturated and polyunsaturated). Sugars and processed carbohydrates joined the prohibited list and after a couple of weeks, complex carbohydrates were limited to just one serve per day. Within one month my diet comprised nothing but fruit and vegetables. In hindsight, this was nowhere near enough for normal daily activity and far too restrictive for the amount of exercise I was doing. My body needed protein. It longed for fat. It craved complex carbohydrates. But they were the enemy and although my stomach grumbled, I refused to give in. I went to bed with hunger pains, but I learned to ignore them.

In addition to restricting my kilojoule intake, I kept up a strict exercise regime. I ran the same route every day to ensure I covered exactly twelve kilometres; not one metre less. Missing a session was not an option, either. I trained rain, hail or shine. In addition to running, I cycled and walked an hour each day.

'I think you're overdoing it,' my mother said to me one morning as she sat at the kitchen table eating her cereal while I put on my running shoes.

'What are you talking about?' I replied shortly. 'It's healthy to exercise.'

'Yes, I agree,' she said. 'But in moderation.'

'I'm not doing that much. Many people run every day and I cycle to get to work. What's wrong with that?'

'I'm just worried about you, that's all,' replied Mum, nervously scratching her hair.

'Please don't worry,' I said. I hugged her and headed out the door for my run. I knew deep down that I was doing too much but I tried to justify it to myself: a daily twelve kilometre run is not excessive; cycling was my mode of transport and a one hour walk could only be healthy. Couldn't it?

No-one ever mentioned the words 'eating disorder' or 'exercise addiction' and although a part of me could feel myself falling into the depths of both, I would never have admitted it to anyone. I was aware of athletic anorexia, a condition characterised by exercise addiction and an obsession with maintaining a low body weight, but I refused to believe I fitted that description.

I was in denial and convinced myself that because I knew I wasn't fat – I was happy with my body and just determined to maintain it – there was nothing wrong. Moreover, my determined, dominating nature, supported by what I now describe as the delusional voice in my head, wasn't about to relinquish control. I became so self-absorbed, so distracted by my obsession with keeping track of every kilojoule I consumed and expended, that I was unaware that I had veered onto a path to self-destruction. I was also so focused on not relinquishing control of my body, that I misinterpreted any comments my parents or Brent made about my weight and my eating or exercise habits, oblivious to the fact that they were only trying to help me. I wasn't prepared to listen to anyone. Except, that is, for my new companion, the voice.

5

2005   Dangerously disciplined

It was the beginning of April 2005, three months since I had returned from overseas, back to the monotony of running, work and life. I was still in Melbourne living with my parents and Brent was living with his parents. Neither of us were sure whether we wanted to remain in Melbourne or live overseas again. I lay on my bed in the room in which I grew up, staring at the photos of family and friends that covered the walls and then at the numerous sporting trophies decorating the shelves. They represented success; I had excelled and proven that I was the best on the day. I glanced at a photo taken at my high school formal and was shocked to see how big I looked and how chubby my cheeks were, a reminder of how I looked when I was heavier. I rolled over and reached for the latest edition of *Runner's World* magazine on my bedside table. I bought the magazine, which included useful running articles such as how to increase your speed and how to adopt a runner's body, every month. I was constantly in awe of the models sprawled across the front cover, their athletic bodies with defined six packs and long, athletic legs that most can only dream of. I loved the toned look and have always had a desire to be tall. At five foot three inches or one hundred and sixty-one centimetres, there wasn't much I could do to change my height, but the past couple of years had proved that I could be in control of my body shape.

An advertisement on the first page captured my attention. *Runner's World* was holding a competition to be part of the Nike

Running Team in the lead-up to the Melbourne Marathon. I read the details. Steve Moneghetti was to coach the team. The selected runners would be flown to New Zealand for a training camp, including fitness testing at Auckland University. Monaghetti would prescribe an individualised training program based on each runner's goals and current fitness level. Nike would sponsor the team for the months leading up to the race, with all running gear provided. The team were to stay in a hotel in Melbourne the weekend of the race and be driven by bus to the start line.

Wow, I thought. This is exactly what I need to escape the monotony of my training. And it might force me to start fuelling my body properly. Running the same twelve-kilometre route every day at the same pace had become tedious and my recent obsession over counting kilojoules and exercising excessively left me little time for much else. I avoided social gatherings, not only for fear of relinquishing discipline but because I didn't have much energy, and this was also beginning to take a toll on my relationship with Brent.

'You're always out running,' he said to me one afternoon when he rang and asked if he could come and see me. 'You never have time for me any more.'

'That's not true,' was all I could manage. 'I run once or twice a day, that's it.'

'How about I come over tonight and cook you dinner?' he suggested. 'Then we can go to see a movie.'

'You don't have to do that,' I replied. 'How about you just come over after dinner and we can watch TV? I'm too tired to go out.'

I didn't realise it at the time but my response confirmed what Brent had just said. I was too tired to go to the movies, having spent all the energy I had running. And I didn't want Brent cooking me dinner because that would mean I wouldn't have total control of what went into the meal.

I was significantly smaller than my fifty-four kilogram build two years earlier, but I had been happier then. I desperately needed something to help me find a healthy balance; to return to eating well and exercising for the goal of good health and another successful marathon. Being a part of this team was exactly the opportunity I needed. A complimentary Nike wardrobe wouldn't hurt, either. As part of the application process, I had to write in less than 100 words why I should be chosen for Team Nike. I was ashamed to expose the real truth, so this is what I wrote.

'I ran a 3:07 marathon last year but my training has since become stale and I have reached a plateau. My next goal is to run under three hours but I know in order to do this I need expert advice on my training program and diet. I believe that with the correct guidance and support, I will be able to achieve my goal and break three hours for the Melbourne Marathon.'

The magazine asked you to include a photograph of yourself. I attached the most attractive photograph I could find (a nice smile can go a long way) and put my application in the mail the same day. At work that afternoon I overheard someone talking about the Nike Running Team advertisement.

'It sounds great,' he said to his friend. 'I'm definitely going to apply. But I heard they're only selecting a team of eight runners from all around Australia and New Zealand.'

The following morning my alarm sounded at 6 am, as it did every morning. Recently the light on the alarm had begun to glow more strongly as the mornings got darker and my nose felt colder; the warmth of the bed was even harder to leave. The Melbourne winter was fast approaching, and some mornings were filled with mist. Maximum temperatures had plummeted to the low teens over the past few weeks and overnight temperatures were in single digits. As I had done for a couple of months, I woke up feeling fatigued and lethargic. I wanted nothing more than to roll over and go back to sleep but I knew if I did, I would regret it for the entire day. I would be ridden with guilt for not expending the usual one-thousand kilojoules before work. The voice in my head spurred me on to drag myself out of bed and switch on the light, my eyes half open. My legs felt heavy and sore. My eyes stung with fatigue, but I was not about to give in and crawl back into bed. Think about how good you will feel in an hour, I tried to convince myself.

But deep down I knew I would feel far from great. After months of running the same distance at the same pace, I no longer felt the endorphins and didn't finish with a runner's high. All I felt was an extreme low if I didn't run, my solemn mood making me far-from-pleasant company for others. I would also feel undeserving of food.

With this thought firmly engraved in my conscience, I pulled on my yellow crop top and a purple long-sleeved, dri-fit top and navy full-length leggings. With my eyes still half closed, next I put on my socks and shoes. Then my white cap to keep my long, thick plait out of my face. Lastly my running gloves to prevent my fingers feeling the morning chill and going numb. I tiptoed quietly out the back door, cautious not to wake my parents. I was glad they were both still asleep as I didn't want to talk to anyone before I ran. I just wanted to get out the door, run my twelve kilometres and return home. Only then did I feel ready to begin my day.

The run was no different to usual. I felt terrible for the first three kilometres before I found my rhythm and the lead-like feeling in my legs began to dissipate. When I got home I had a shower and ate breakfast. Although I had earned the right to eat, I was still careful with my choice; adamant not to consume more kilojoules than I had expended. I opted for the usual bowl of fruit, ignoring the fact that the kilojoules it provided equated to no more than a four-kilometre run. I was still a little hungry when I finished but I shut down the temptation to eat more. Control. Don't give in. I prepared my lunch and snacks for the day – a banana, an apple, a plum, a handful of strawberries and a small bunch of grapes – and got ready to cycle to work.

I had cycled to work every day for the past five years. I had ridden in forty-degree heat in the midst of the Melbourne summer, with sweat mixing in with the grime of the city air leaving a film on my skin. I had survived eighty per cent humidity in North Queensland, arriving at work saturated with sweat, having to peel the clothes off my skin. On numerous occasions I had ridden through a blanket of fog as the Melbourne sun attempted to pierce the thick haze. There were trips to work in downpour, my vision blurred by the sheets of rain. But worst of all were the gusty winds hurling towards me at alarming speeds, requiring greater strength than tackling a steep hill.

This particular morning was cold but not freezing. I put on my thick woollen gloves and my charcoal grey backpack before mounting my bike and riding down our driveway. I really can't be bothered, I thought. Why don't I just drive like most people would if they felt like this? The voice in my head reminded me why driving wasn't an option: cycling was another chance to burn kilojoules. If I surrendered, I would feel guilty for the whole day. A sensible (but weak and timid) voice tried to rationalise and tell me that this was a ludicrous way of thinking.

I knew that. I wasn't stupid. But the other more powerful voice asked me how I could even consider driving. 'Don't be so lazy,' it screamed at me. 'Just ride. Get on the bike and start pedalling.' I arrived at work forty minutes later, proud that I had not given in and comforted by the fact that I had expended more energy. And I had no choice but to ride home at the end of the day.

I was going for my nightly walk after a busy day at work when my phone rang. 'Vanessa?' said the lady on the other end of the phone.

'Yes, speaking,' I replied.

'This is Bridget from Nike. I am ringing to inform you that you have been chosen to be part of Team Nike.' I hesitated for a couple of seconds, not sure I had heard correctly.

'Are you serious?' was all I could manage.

'Yes, your application has been successful. Congratulations. I just want to confirm that you would still like to be part of the team.'

'Yes, yes of course,' I blurted out. 'Wow, I'm shocked. Thank you so much.'

'You are required to attend a training camp in Auckland, New Zealand in three weeks. Will you be available?' Bridget asked me.

'Yes, of course,' I said without giving it any thought. 'I can't wait.'

'Great,' she replied. 'We are very happy to have you on board. I will email you some information about the camp and your inclusion in Team Nike. There will be a phone conference with team members and your coach, Steve Moneghetti, next Wednesday.'

Steve Moneghetti? The Steve Moneghetti? He really was going to coach me? Wow, this was a dream come true. I hung up the phone, bursting with jubilation. I was one of eight people from

Australia and New Zealand who had been chosen to be part of Team Nike! I hung up the phone and immediately rang Brent. His reaction was more enthusiastic than I had expected, after he had recently told me my running was leaving little time for our relationship. But he knew how much I loved running and what it would mean to me if I did break three hours in the marathon.

'Great job, hun! That's awesome. You'll be running faster than me soon,' he joked.

'Thanks! I'm really excited. And I promise my running won't get in the way of us from now on,' I reassured him. I'm not sure how convincing I sounded, especially because I wasn't convinced myself, but he congratulated me once again.

I hung up from Brent and ran home, taking a short cut through the park, past the myriad of laughing children playing on the playground. When I arrived home I burst through the front door and flung it wide open. It slammed against the wall as I ran inside and straight to the kitchen where Mum was busy preparing dinner and Dad was laying plates and cutlery on the dining table. They both looked up as soon as I entered, startled at my sudden entrance.

'Guess what?' I cried. 'I've been selected to be part of Team Nike. I'm going to New Zealand in three weeks. Steve Moneghetti will be my coach. I'm going to get lots of free Nike clothes.'

I caught my breath and waited nervously for their response. I knew my parents would be thrilled for me, but I also knew they would be worried that this would only motivate me to train harder. They made no secret of the fact they didn't like me running marathons.

'They are not good for you,' Mum had said on several occasions.

'Humans are not designed to run so far.'

In fact, during my first marathon in Townsville my parents were so worried I would collapse, they asked a friend of mine to call them during the race with updates on my progress. Because the route had involved three loops of the same route, my friend saw me approximately every hour and called each time to reassure them I was running well.

So when I broke the news of my Team Nike selection, their response wasn't surprising. As always, they demonstrated their full support with a hug and kiss, but expressed caution.

'Congratulations,' they both said, almost simultaneously.

'But please be careful,' my mum added. 'You are too precious to me.'

14 May 2005

I have been chosen for Team Nike! I am so excited, I've been on a high since I received the call yesterday afternoon. Free Nike clothes, expert training advice from Steve Moneghetti, a man I have previously only seen on television. I'm going to be monitored by a sports dietician, a podiatrist, an exercise physiologist. This is a dream come true! But I know I'm going to have to change my current lifestyle. Successful athletes don't train with the intention of burning as many kilojoules as possible. They do not think, 'I'd better not eat too much or I might put on weight'. I'm going to have to change my mindset and that means battling the voice inside my head. It's not going to be easy but I'm determined! From now on I am going to eat and train to become faster and fitter. And healthier.

6

Enter denial

In June I flew to Auckland, New Zealand, where I met Team Nike and our coach, Steve Moneghetti. The group's running abilities and personal best times varied, with two runners training for their first marathon. A Nike bag filled with running gear and several pairs of running shoes awaited us when we entered our hotel rooms. It smelt like a miniature chemical factory, with the strong but enticing odour of the new shoes impossible to ignore, but it felt like Christmas. Crop tops, long-sleeve tops, and running shorts of different colours lit up the room. Next to them lay several Nike caps, pairs of socks, drink bottles and towels.

During the four days we underwent numerous fitness tests including a VO2 max test to measure our cardiovascular endurance – the ability of the body to consume and utilise oxygen to produce energy – and a biomechanical analysis to help determine which Nike shoe best suited our foot type. I was advised to wear the Nike Zoom Elite shoe. My high mileage meant I would need a new pair every six to eight weeks. Running shoes are expensive, so I was extremely grateful to be given a few pairs.

We each had a private consultation with a sports dietician. Karen was a woman of no more than thirty, slim and glamorous, with long wavy red hair and dark brown eyes. She seemed friendly. She asked me to complete a food diary representing my dietary intake for the past week. I confess that what I wrote was not one hundred per cent true. I was embarrassed to reveal my far-from-adequate diet so I added a bowl of cereal to each breakfast and a sandwich to each lunch. Even with these additions, she told me I needed to increase my carbohydrate and fat intake. Imagine if I had told her the truth, I thought.

Karen then wrote me an eating plan. Not a strict diet but rather a list of suggestions for each meal as well as morning and afternoon snacks. Well aware that I should have been following a similar plan all along, I was not surprised by any of her recommendations. In fact, my consultation with Karen confirmed what I already knew: if I wanted to make the most of this unbelievable opportunity, it was time to stop counting every kilojoule that entered my mouth. I needed to regard food as an essential ingredient for my body rather than a threat to putting on weight. It was truly difficult to believe, though.

Steve Moneghetti wrote me a training program, which totalled a slightly greater weekly mileage than what I was currently doing, but he removed the present monotony. Rather than covering the same distance at the same pace every day, my program included two interval sessions (eight times four hundred metres and five times one kilometre), a tempo run (fifteen to twenty kilometres at race pace – the pace at which I was hoping to run the marathon) and a long run (starting at twenty-five kilometres and building to thirty-eight kilometres over a couple of months). In addition, I would do two to three easy runs of ten to twelve kilometres and a couple of short runs of six kilometres. I wasn't thrilled about the interval sessions, but I knew that they would make me run faster.

I felt a zest and motivation for training that I hadn't experienced in a long time. I was impatient to begin my new program and decided to approach it the only way I knew how: with sheer determination and will. I would run the Melbourne Marathon in under three hours.

Mr Stevens was a short, stocky man in his early sixties. With a grey moustache and small, silver-rimmed glasses perched on the end of his nose, he resembled a professor. He had been a secondary school physics teacher and had excelled as a four-hundred-metre runner, representing Australia on numerous occasions. He had coached many school athletics teams and individual endurance female athletes, so he was well aware of common issues faced by females in this field. It was for this reason that Megan, the receptionist at my work, suggested I see him.

Initially, I was reluctant. I was being coached by one of Australia's greatest marathoners of all time and didn't feel the need for any extra support or mentoring. Instead, I continued to insist that running was just a hobby that helped to relieve stress and keep me in shape. But what I didn't realise was that to everyone around me, it was very clear that running had evolved into a dangerous pursuit.

Megan had confided that she had been forced out of competitive running from overtraining, and was adamant that I meet with Mr Stevens. Trusting her opinion, I agreed. I had no idea what we were going to talk about and because he had never seen me run, I wondered how he'd be able to help me. Nonetheless, I was looking forward to our meeting. Instinctively, I knew I needed support.

Three weeks after my trip to New Zealand, one grey, dreary Sunday afternoon, I met Mr Stevens at a quiet suburban café. I spotted him immediately, recognising him from his description of himself over the phone. I walked over to the table where he sat sipping a coffee, white froth forming on his moustache with each sip. He was reading the sports section of the local newspaper.

'Mr Stevens?' I asked. He nodded and signalled for me to sit down opposite him. 'It's nice to meet you,' I said as I shook his hand.

'Likewise,' he replied. I put my new red Nike backpack on the floor, which held my water bottle, wallet and keys. I sat down on the blue chair in front of him, unsure of what to say – there was an air of mystery about him as he assessed me with cold, glazed eyes, analysing my every movement. This did nothing to ease my nerves.

'Would you like a drink or something to eat?' he asked.

'No thanks,' I replied without hesitation. 'I just ate and I have my water here.' I pointed to my water bottle, which I carried everywhere.

Bad mistake, I thought. Now he probably thinks I don't eat. During the past year, whenever I refused food, I sensed that people judged me and assumed I had an eating disorder. I was wearing my skinny jeans and knew I looked thin, but I was a marathon runner, after all. Endurance runners are not supposed to carry any fat.

Mr Stevens ordered a chicken baguette with a glass of coke. A part of me wanted to order the same, but the voice in my head made sure I refrained. 'Too much sugar and too many carbs. You've only run twelve kilometres this morning. That doesn't qualify for a baguette that big.' I was hungry, but I knew the feeling would pass.

'So I hear you're a pretty good runner,' Mr Stevens started.

What was I meant to say to that? Yeah, I'm great. I'm awesome. 'Not bad,' I replied.

The air was tense. I could feel the awkwardness and wished I hadn't agreed to meet him. I didn't even consider myself a good runner – I had only run three marathons and although I had improved quite significantly with each race, I was a long way off from qualifying for the elite category. I felt compelled to stand up, thank him and tell him not to waste any more of his time. Yet I was intrigued as to what he might say and how he could help me.

'Do you have a training program?' he asked.

'Yes, I am being coached by Steve Moneghetti. He's devised my program,' I replied proudly, going on to describe my training schedule in detail.

'How are your four-hundred-metre sessions going?' he asked.

'Terribly,' I said, the enthusiasm draining from me. 'I hate them and I can't do them. I'm not a track runner,' I admitted, defeatedly.

'I'd like to watch you do a session at some stage,' he said. 'I want to have a look at your running technique.'

'Sure,' I replied, grateful that someone else was taking an interest.

'What about your diet?' he asked. 'Do you think you get enough kilojoules each day?'

It was the question I had been dreading. The question I knew I couldn't avoid. Why, oh why does everyone have to bring that up? I couldn't admit the truth. I was a health professional, ashamed of my own tenacious compulsion to train hard while denying my body adequate nourishment. Each day I went to battle with the dominating voice in my head that insisted I count every kilojoule that entered my mouth. Yet each day I surrendered again and continued to obey its demands. Mr Stevens was asking a simple question, but I interpreted it to be threatening. Still in denial, I took offence to his question.

'Yes of course,' I replied abruptly. 'I eat very well and I'm very healthy.'

It was a response I would find myself repeating endlessly over the next couple of years as I faced the same question. I could tell by his reaction that he didn't believe me, but he didn't say anything. He had seen many other female athletes depriving their bodies of essential nutrients, overpowered by an urge to stay lean, so my response wouldn't have shocked him. I went on to explain the consultation I had with the dietician in New Zealand and what she had advised, hoping this would convince him that my diet didn't require further attention.

I remained in touch with Mr Stevens for a few weeks and he accompanied me on a couple of track sessions. Some of his advice was valuable, but when I think back to our conversations, all that remains etched in my memory is the endless questions he asked me about my weight and my diet. In hindsight, he was trying to help me, but I felt vulnerable as he exposed my delusional, troubled self. The self I didn't want anyone to meet. The self I wanted to hide from the outside world.

After a few weeks, I stopped returning his calls, and I haven't spoken to him since.

Brent and I had been back in Melbourne a little less than six months when we decided to head north again. Melbourne's cold, often wet and unpredictable winter weather was not ideal for training. The streets often ran with water and I have memories of finishing a run with my shoes wet and my fingers numb, which made our decision to move to the Sunshine Coast an easy one.

I found a job at a physiotherapy clinic in Maroochydore, situated on a river and across the road from a park and the local swimming pool. It was not far from where Brent owned a small studio apartment, which became our home for four months. It was only a few years old and the floral bed cover and picture frames, typical of hotel decor, gave us the feeling we were on holiday. With the ocean at our doorstep and a running track across the road following the length of the beach, it provided a perfect location for training. The salty smell of the ocean followed me on every run, its spray inviting as it cooled me down and provided some relief from the warmer days. Immersing my legs in the ice-cold, often calm ocean water was the ideal way to recover from long runs and intense interval sessions.

I soon settled into my routine of running and working, while Brent spent time trading on the stock market. Nine training sessions per week in between full-time work left little time or energy for much else but because Brent and I were living together, it felt as though we were spending ample time together again. Brent occasionally joined me on my runs and we fitted in a weekly massage and a night out for dinner on weekends. But most Saturday nights I was in bed by 9.30 pm, in order to prepare for my Sunday morning long runs. These started at 5.30 am to ensure I was finished by 8.30 am, when the sun was out with full force. This was followed by a swim in the ocean and a healthy breakfast. I had worked hard to change my thinking since my consultation with the dietician in New Zealand, and had added a big bowl of cereal and yogurt to my usual fruit. The rest of the day would be spent lazing around the apartment or walking along the beach, conserving energy in preparation for my ten-kilometre run in the evening. For the first few weeks Brent didn't comment on my training, nor did he say anything that suggested he wasn't happy with our set up and he seemed content with our relatively non-eventful weekends. Reluctantly, in addition to my more substantial breakfast, I had begun eating bread for lunch and a small bowl of either rice or pasta for dinner. I had gained a couple of kilograms as a result, which I was very aware of when I pulled on my lycra running shorts. Although I felt heavier, at forty-eight kilograms, I knew I still had very little body fat and constantly reminded myself that I was healthier than I had been a few months earlier.

I followed my training program religiously and was happy to report my progress to coach Moneghetti (aka Mona) and team Nike during our fortnightly teleconferences. Mona was amazed at my discipline. I clocked every training session using my Nike watch and downloaded the times onto my computer. I was motivated by the improvements in my interval sessions as well as my tempo and long runs. My long runs peaked at thirty-eight kilometres six weeks out from the Melbourne Marathon, after which we were advised to start tapering to ensure we felt fresh on the day of the race.

I completed every training session during the week alone so I could run exactly when and where I wanted. Selfish, I know, but I didn't have time to waste waiting for people and fitting in to others' schedules. Occasionally Brent joined me for parts of my long runs, as did a few runners who I met out on the track. I told them where I would be at approximately what time and if they were there, I was happy for them to join me, provided they ran at my pace. If they weren't, I wouldn't wait for them.

I wasn't aware at the time of how selfish and self-absorbed I had become. I spoke to my best friend, Anna, on the phone once a week and occasionally I was in contact with other friends back in Melbourne, but apart from work colleagues and the odd runner I met out on the running track, I made no effort to make new friends and failed to recognise how isolated I had become. Just as a lone bird glides through the sky, I pounded the footpath for mile after mile, single-minded, focused only on putting one foot in front of the other, oblivious to the world going on around me. Running was my preoccupation. No-one and nothing else mattered.

'Shall we go out for dinner tonight?' Brent asked one Saturday evening, about two months after we had moved to the Coast. I had been working all day at the clinic and was absolutely exhausted.

'Sorry, I don't feel like it tonight,' I replied instantly, making it clear I wouldn't even consider it. 'It's been a long week. I need an early night so I'm ready for my long run in the morning.'

'We haven't been out for so long,' Brent said, a slight whine in his voice. 'Not even for dinner. You just run and work and do nothing else.' I didn't even look up from my book that I was reading to notice his slouched shoulders or his dejected face. I chose to ignore the note of despair in his voice. 'That's not true,' I said, refusing to meet his gaze, scared of the truth and highlighting the growing distance between us.

'Yes it is. From the moment you wake up, you're out the door running. You come home, have breakfast, go straight to work, train again when you get home from work, eat dinner and go to bed. We don't spend any quality time together anymore. We don't have fun like we used to. And I can't remember the last time you showed me any affection. The worst thing is, you are so caught up in it all that you don't even realise all this. You can't even see how your training is taking over our lives.' He began to speak more quickly, the volume of his voice increasing. Brent very rarely raised his voice or displayed anger but when I noticed his knuckles turning white, gripping the glass he was holding, I finally looked up and met his gaze. His infuriation and frustration were building; he was using every bit of energy to stop himself exploding. At the same time he looked upset, almost defeated, as if he didn't know what else to do or say to change my ways and save our relationship. I knew what he was saying was true, but I was unable to reach him, to acknowledge what was destroying me – and us.

'Hun, I work hard and yes my training is important at the moment. You need to understand that.' I realised even as I said it that my call for empathy was hollow, barely hiding the truth that I was struggling to deny.

'I do understand, but it's become an obsession. Something has got to change or we're not going to last.' With that Brent placed his glass on the table and walked out, slamming the door behind him. He went out for dinner on his own. This hostility was new to me and left me speechless. I knew if I didn't want to lose him I desperately had to change my lifestyle but wasn't sure how to go about it. I had a shower, ate a salad, set my alarm for 5 am and went to bed, wondering how I could get myself out of this cobweb I had become entangled in.

7

The dream run

I continued to keep a training log and jot down feelings in my diary leading up to the Melbourne Marathon. I recorded how I felt during my runs, after each run and outside of running, in the hope that this would help to untangle the confusion in my mind.

8 October 2005

We came down to Melbourne a few days ago. So great to see family and friends again. I'm feeling confident leading up to Sunday but right now I'm feeling fat and lazy. I've only run thirty kilometres this week! I keep telling myself it's for the best, so I feel fresh and ready to go on Sunday. I just want the day to arrive! Brent and I have had our moments the past few weeks but I've assured him I will reduce my training after the Melbourne Marathon is over. I know I've been difficult to live with and my running has taken over a bit but it's hard not to concentrate all my energy towards the big race. Only two days to go!

Brent and I stayed in a hotel the night before of the Melbourne Marathon. The other members of Team Nike stayed there, too. We woke up the morning of the race to a cold, wet, windy day. I remember sodden leaves in the wet gutters as we boarded the bus, the wind moaning and rustling heavily through the desolate trees. This was not the weather I had been hoping for. I got dressed in my Nike running gear: navy lycra running shorts and fluorescent yellow crop top, a pair of white socks and my white racing shoes with a gold Nike tick embroidered on the side – my uniform for every long run the past three months. I put on a pair of track pants and two jackets over the top, proud to display the Nike logo. I packed my running gloves and cap in my bag and headed to the foyer of the hotel to meet the rest of Team Nike.

Brent had entered the half marathon. He kissed me warmly and wished me luck before making his way to the city centre to board his bus to the start line, which was situated at the halfway mark of the full marathon. I returned the kiss and wished him good luck also, feeling my emotion building, aware of how much he had put up with the past few months and how distant I had become. Since he had stormed out that Saturday evening, I had promised him that after the Melbourne Marathon life would return to normal – running would no longer be my priority and I would find the time (and energy) for our relationship. I'm not sure he was entirely convinced, as his sole response was a nod of the head as he said 'We'll see.' I proceeded to board my bus.

I sat alone, preferring not to talk to anyone. As we were driven to the start line, the rain trickled down the grimy window, leaving tracks of clear glass. I stared through them and visualised the race. I concentrated hard on the vision of myself running effortlessly, feeling strong and crossing the finish line with the clock displaying a time – any time – under three hours.

Halfway into the thirty-minute drive, Mona came and sat next to me. He asked me how I was feeling.

'A bit nervous,' I replied. 'But okay.'

He fixed his eyes on mine. 'You'll be fine once the gun goes off,' he replied, a tone of certainty and reassurance in his voice. 'You know you have put in all the hard work. Just see this race as another Sunday long run. Ignore everyone around you and go out at your own pace.'

This was the best piece of advice he could have given me. I knew what pace I needed to run in order to break three hours and I was also aware that to break three hours, I would most likely have to run a negative split, meaning the second half of the race would have to be faster than the first.

'Have you had breakfast?' Mona asked as he watched me nibble away at half an energy bar.

'Just this,' I replied.

'That's not enough. You need to eat more.' A look of concern crossed his face. I knew he was right but I also knew that I had survived every long run for the past three months on half an energy bar.

'No, it's okay,' I said. 'It's all I ever eat before a long run. I don't want to do anything differently.'

He was content with my response, aware of the importance of following the same routine as during training. I knew myself that half an energy bar was not actually enough before a long run, but I didn't want to start the day with any more kilojoules – it would leave me fewer 'allowed' kilojoules for the rest of the day. And I had made it through my long runs before, so why change now?

Mona continued on his way down the bus to talk to the other runners. I returned my intense focus to the race. I finished my energy bar and although I felt a little peckish, I knew the feeling would pass, just as it did before every long run.

As I stood on the start line, nerves began to take over my body. I could feel my heart pounding, my stomach churning. The sky was dark, the air in front of my face turned to mist as I breathed out and rain continued to fall lightly. I had removed my outer layers of clothing and was wearing only my lycra running shorts and crop top revealing a six pack of muscle and my twig-like arms. I kept my gloves on to keep my hands warm. I felt freezing from head to toe and I could feel the moisture in my shoes. The temperature was less than half of what I was used to in Queensland. Glancing around me I noticed that no-one seemed to be shivering like I was. Most runners were wearing shorts and t-shirts, while some had singlets and a few women were wearing crop tops but I spotted only one other person with gloves on. I tried to keep my legs moving to prevent them from stiffening up. I looked at my watch to make sure I had set it properly. Suddenly the countdown was on and then ...

'On your marks, get set ... BANG!'

I found myself in the zone after three kilometres. I glanced at my watch – 12 minutes 30 seconds. I was on track. I just needed to maintain my pace for another thirty-nine kilometres and my goal would be accomplished.

I found myself running with a group of about ten runners. As I took in the lithe, sinewy bodies around me, the number and sponsors flapping on their shirts, I realised I was the only female in the pack. A handful of females had gone out faster than me, but I erased this from my mind. I wasn't there to win the race or even finish in the top five. I was there to race against myself, to run a personal best time and break three hours.

Some runners like to talk while they are running and I caught snippets of previous marathon experiences. Words were spoken on the exhale, a few at a time, in shorthand, but I tuned out, intent on remaining focused and losing myself in the immensity of the race. Scott, a representative from Nike, asked me before the race if I'd mind if he ran alongside me. I didn't, but I warned him I wouldn't want to engage in conversation.

As an elite marathon runner, Scott totally understood. The only words we exchanged were when he occasionally asked me how I was feeling. I replied at a minimum, refusing to take my eyes off the road ahead of me. A couple of times he ordered me to slow down, aware that I had unintentionally increased my speed to a pace that I most likely wouldn't be able to maintain.

I tucked in behind two men, the brands on the back of their sneakers bobbing up and down with each step. The headwind gained in ferocity, forcing me to push forward with greater strength and threatening to add several minutes to my time. As we approached the halfway mark the road became a gradual uphill slope; not what my increasingly tight calves were hoping for. I kept my focus, making sure to maintain my rhythm and remain 'in the zone' Towards the halfway mark, a few runners in the pack began to wane. Before long, only five of us remained. Other than my calves, I felt great and found the pace comfortable. As we passed the twenty-one-kilometre mark, I looked down at my watch, which was wet from the rain that continued to fall lightly. One hour thirty minutes. If I could run a negative split, I would break three hours. At around the thirty-kilometre mark, three runners dropped off, leaving Scott and I running alone.

'How are you feeling?' he asked, wiping the sweat from his brow.

'Great,' I replied, ignoring the knives digging into every muscle in my legs. My state of mind would be pivotal in whether I reached my goal. I had to block out the pain that was beginning to engulf my body.

Come on, I urged myself, more determined than ever. Only twelve kilometres to go. That's no more than a standard daily run. I knew I had the mental strength to do it, to complete the race in under three hours. I felt more determined that ever. I was just hoping, praying that my body was in sync with my mind. I could hear the crowd cheering in rhythmic pattern from the side of the road, tape flapping between us. At the thirty-four-kilometre mark I noticed three female runners ahead of me, ponytails swishing and elbows swaying. I was closing in on them without increasing my pace. They are hurting, I thought. I can catch them.

A few minutes later, I passed their brightly coloured tank tops. I overtook another two females at the thirty-eight-kilometre mark and was hurting all over, but the adrenaline had well and truly kicked in. I could feel it coursing through my body, making my veins bulge and deafening me with its whirr in my head at the same time. At the thirty-nine-kilometre mark, I caught a glimpse of Mona, his trademark effortless and fluent running style easy to recognise. He was running alongside the fastest male runner in Team Nike, whose goal had been to run under two hours forty-five minutes, but from his short, shuffled steps, sweaty hands slipping on his hips, and his elevated shoulders, it was evident he was struggling.

As I glided past them, I heard Mona yell out, 'Go Vanessa.'

I glanced at my watch, the glass face glistening in the emerging sunshine, and knew then that I would secure my place firmly in the exclusive sub-three-hour marathon club. Pain was ravaging every muscle in my legs but I have never felt stronger or more powerful than at that moment. Boosted by some latent adrenaline and the raucous cheer from the crowd that seemed to swell as I passed, I felt like I was on a world stage as I went up another gear at the forty-kilometre mark. My foot planted firmly on the accelerator, I entered the home straight and ran the last kilometre faster than any other I had run that day.

I crossed the finish line in third place with a time of 2:54.11. I heard the squeals of my best friend Anna, herself an elite four-hundred metre runner, who was waiting at the finish line. I ran straight into the secure arms of my family, their strength and embraces lifting me up, and I struggled to hold back tears as I hugged Brent, who had finished his half marathon an hour earlier. Anna later told me that she relived the moment I crossed the line over and over, and this inspired her during her training sessions. What I felt at that moment is indescribable and something I will cherish forever. The hard training had paid off – as had the small, but important, changes I had made to my lifestyle. I still had a long way to go to achieve a healthy balance, but those extra daily kilojoules had been worth it.

It was by far the best moment of my life.

The months leading up to the Melbourne Marathon had been filled with such excitement and anticipation. How fast could I run and how good could I be? The build-up had been intense and with the single focus required, it had taken over my life – and Brent's. With the race now over, I returned to the Sunshine Coast while Brent decided to return to Thailand to work for six months. He assured me his decision had nothing to do with my excessive training and that he still wanted to maintain our relationship, but for now it was the right move for work. Although we remained a couple,

I found myself suddenly on my own, and with no immediate goal to train for.

It takes a good few months to fully recover from a marathon, both mentally and physically and I was expecting to suffer some post-race blues. I missed doing my regular Sunday long runs, but I couldn't entertain the thought of training for another marathon anytime soon, so I took two months off my strict training schedule, exchanging my regime with regular, short runs and swimming. The seventy kilometres a week I was now running was far less than what I had been covering during the previous months.

Following my effort at the Melbourne Marathon, a few coaches expressed an interest in coaching me. I had planned to keep in touch with Mona, but he was always only going to coach Team Nike during the lead-up to the Melbourne Marathon. Scott Nicholas, the Nike representative who had run with me during the race, was my obvious choice. We had gotten to know each other the days leading up to the race and during the race. He had respected my wish not to engage in any conversation during the marathon and had slowed me down at appropriate times. I felt like he could help take me to the next level – to another personal best time.

Scott was an American living in Melbourne and had marginally missed out on the US Olympic team in 2004 with a personal best time of 2:18. He was of medium height, lean, with wavy brown hair and an ever-present smile. I was impressed by his calm, positive nature, his optimistic attitude and his unwavering belief that you can achieve anything you set your mind to. I loved his never-say-die attitude, and his encouragement during the Melbourne Marathon had been instrumental to my success. We agreed the coach/athlete relationship could work despite living two-thousand kilometres from each other.

We agreed to meet whenever I was back in Melbourne and communicate regularly by phone. We devised a race schedule for the following twelve months which included two marathons, a couple of half marathons and a few shorter races (five and ten kilometres). Having never been a track runner, the short races were an important aspect of my training if I wanted to improve my speed and achieve another personal best time.

My first five-kilometre race, the Noosa Bolt, was one month after the Melbourne Marathon. It was a curtain-raiser to the famous Noosa Triathlon and attracted an elite field, requiring a qualifying time of under twenty minutes. They disqualified you from the race if you failed to complete the first half in under ten minutes. I knew the calibre of runners would be out of my league, but Scott believed it would be a great experience lining up against the country's best.

As I stood at the start line, I felt overwhelmed by the talent standing alongside me. The display of lean, athletic physiques of well-known Olympians and Commonwealth Games medallists, including Mona, Craig Mottram, Kerryn McCann and Sonia O'Sullivan was intimidating. This is a fantastic experience, I tried to convince myself. Enjoy it and learn from it.

I began the race with two goals in mind: to avoid disqualification at the halfway mark and not to finish last. I ran the first kilometre faster than I had ever run a kilometre before – only to find myself in last position. To have run my heart out, faster than I thought possible, only to find myself in last position was not just disheartening, it was embarrassing. Lactic acid had consumed my body and there were still four kilometres to go.

Thankfully I crossed the halfway mark in just under 9 minutes and 30 seconds, so I was allowed to continue. Still in last position, I was boosted to the finish by thousands of raucous, cheering spectators, waving their arms about and screaming at the top of their lungs. I crossed the finish line in 19.20. I had pushed my body to the absolute limit and felt worse physically than I had at the end of the Melbourne Marathon.

The race confirmed what I already knew: I needed to work on my speed and increase my anaerobic threshold (the point at which lactic acid takes over your body and forces you to slow down), if I was to going to take my running to the next level. It was time for more interval sessions.

Following my effort in the Melbourne Marathon, I was offered sponsorship with PowerBar. They supplied me with gels, electrolyte drinks, protein powder and energy bars. I was grateful that Nike continued to support me, too, providing me with shoes and clothing. My new training program had me covering approximately one hundred and twenty kilometres per week and considering running shoes should be changed every five to six hundred kilometres, I would have to change shoes every five weeks. This amounted to ten to twelve pairs over the next year. In addition, I needed a pair of racing flats (for speed sessions and races) and track shoes (for my track sessions). Who said running wasn't expensive?

By the beginning of December I felt rested and hungry for more competition. My next goal was to run 2:45 at the Canberra Marathon in April, in four months' time. Scott's program involved nine sessions per week. I trained six days per week and on three days, I did two sessions. Monday was my rest day, but I still walked eight kilometres in the morning. This was not part of my training program, but if I didn't do something I would feel fat and lazy. My Sunday long runs began at twenty-five kilometres and increased rapidly so that by January, I was comfortably covering thirty.

The word 'elite' was mentioned on several occasions to describe me, but I never considered myself worthy of this category. For the majority of elite athletes, sport is their profession. They are the best in the country, sometimes the world, and many are paid to compete. They don't work full time. They have access to physiotherapists, doctors and sport psychologists. I didn't believe I was even close to qualifying for this prestigious label, but I approached my training as though my life depended on it.

8 December 2005

I feel so lonely. Brent is in Thailand, my family and friends are in Melbourne, and other than running and work colleagues, I don't really know anyone up here on the Sunshine Coast. In a way, though, it's exactly how I want my life to be — it allows me to concentrate all my efforts and energy into training. Every day I set my alarm for 6 am or earlier if I'm doing a long run, I throw on my running clothes and I'm out the door in ten minutes. I come home, have a shower, eat breakfast, walk the short three kilometres to work, treat patients all day, walk home, eat dinner and go to bed, ready to repeat it all the following day. Some days I train again after work. But I miss Brent, I really do. The worst is at night, having to go to bed alone. I have so much time to myself, so much time to think. Sometimes I think about the future and what I really

want in life. Can I keep this gruelling routine up forever?
What about when Brent and I are physically together again?
I promised him my running wouldn't get in the way of our
relationship after the Melbourne Marathon. I know if I don't
keep that promise I'll lose him.

My life was routine and mundane. My eating became as rigorous as my running schedule and I quickly fell back into the same restrictive habits as before the Melbourne Marathon. My daily food intake resembled that of a celebrity on the cover of *New Idea*: a bowl of fruit, yogurt and cereal for breakfast, a sandwich and a piece of fruit for lunch and some type of meat with veggies or salad for dinner. I felt tremendous guilt if I ate anything more. Only on Sundays did I allow myself a couple of treats, such as an ice cream and a donut, if I had run for over two hours. I became jealous of women who looked fit and lean without having to exercise to extreme and I envied people who allowed themselves chocolate cake without exercising first. Scott sent me a book for Christmas which provided valuable information on nutrition for athletes – in retrospect I am sure he was concerned about whether I was fuelling my body adequately. Although I took some interest in reading it, I chose to ignore the credible advice it provided.

One morning I just decided to stop eating cereal for breakfast – I didn't think I really needed it – opting for only fruit instead. Despite a few extra hunger pangs, I survived the day and made it through my training sessions so decided I didn't need it from that day on. The following week I eliminated bread from my lunch – I was sure I could do without that too – and replaced it with a salad.

Within a month I had totally eliminated all complex

carbohydrates from my diet and the only sugars I was consuming were from fruit and yogurt. I ignored the lethargic, heavy feeling in my legs at the beginning of each run, convincing myself that my body was taking a while to warm up. I continued to deny it was a sign my petrol tank was running on empty.

If I was invited to a social event, I accepted only if it didn't interfere with my training schedule. If I was tired, I trained. If I was sick, I trained. People commended me on my discipline, unaware that my will and determination to complete every session was less to do with self-discipline and more a reflection of a dangerous obsession. The voice in my head consumed me, and continued to torture me.

As a physiotherapist, I told patients that rest was important in order to allow the body to recover. I was well aware that inadequate rest could be detrimental, but with an elite label attached to my name, I felt pressure to train harder – and most importantly, to maintain the body shape which showed the world that I was a runner.

I lost a couple of kilograms in a few weeks, but I put that down to an increase in my training load. Forty-six kilograms is exactly what the weight of an elite marathon runner should be, I thought. I had no bum and no chest and I loved it. I was in the local paper on numerous occasions, always in my Nike running gear, the lycra hugging my body, my defined abdominals on show. Comments regarding my marathon runner's body were frequent. This only magnified my determination to keep my body fat low.

For a while, things progressed well. I was running faster and becoming fitter. I found myself with spare time after work on Tuesdays and Thursdays so I added a couple of extra sessions to my program. If I trained twice on three days of the week, why couldn't I do the same on four days? Or five? I didn't tell Scott I had increased the number of sessions from nine to eleven as I didn't want to reveal my addiction. Not to him, not to anyone.

Not even to myself.

8

2006 Shattered

Brent and I spoke to each other on the phone regularly. Thailand was three hours behind so during the week we spoke in the evenings and on weekends I called him after I finished training. It was too expensive to call from my mobile phone and I didn't have a home phone so I called from a phone box on the side of the road using an international call card. It was often difficult to hear him, the sound of traffic drowning out our conversation.

During one phone call in the middle of January, Brent mentioned a marathon in Khon Kaen, in the north of Thailand, scheduled the following month. The prize money was three thousand dollars and the previous year's female winning time was over three hours. I told him it sounded great, but that I shouldn't really be racing that distance so soon after the Melbourne Marathon.

'Just consider it another Sunday training run,' he said, optimistically. 'You've never had a bad long run. You won't have to push yourself too hard.'

We both knew that was impossible. In a race situation, the adrenaline kicks in and it is a natural instinct to push that little bit harder.

But there was truth in the fact that I hadn't missed a long run in over a year. I was running thirty to thirty-five kilometres every Sunday so what difference would another seven kilometres make? If I ran the marathon at my usual training pace, I had a good chance of winning. The prize money was attractive, and if I flew to Thailand I could spend time with Brent.

After nearly four months apart, our relationship was beginning to feel the effect of the geographical distance separating us. Our initially daily phone calls had become less frequent and shorter in duration. We rarely told each other we missed each other but spoke robotically about the events of the week. The more time I spent alone, the more self-absorbed and obsessed with running I was becoming. I think we both knew if we didn't see each other soon our relationship might not last.

'You're right,' I replied after much hesitation. 'I'll book my flight tomorrow. I'll see you very soon!'

My departure date was exactly three weeks away. I was excited to be running my first race as a sponsored athlete and spent a happy afternoon ironing on the PowerBar tags to my racing gear in anticipation of the race. The following week I added a ten-kilometre afternoon run to my Sunday morning long run, which was what I had done leading up to the Melbourne Marathon. Although I knew it wasn't the smartest thing to do and in hindsight it was the most imbecilic thing I could have done, it was a good excuse to burn more kilojoules. After all it's advisable to begin reducing your weekly mileage about six weeks out from a race, not increasing it. But I didn't tell Scott and there was no-one else checking on me.

With one week to go I began counting down the days until my departure. I woke up on Sunday morning and jumped out of bed, excited about my last long run before heading to Thailand. I planned on running only twenty-five kilometres, given that there were only seven days before I had to race. After clocking forty-five kilometres the previous Sunday (thirty-five in the morning and ten in the afternoon), I felt a little lazy running such a short distance, but the sensible part of me (although small, there was still a sensible part of me) knew it was the right thing to do.

My runs had become effortless over the past few months, but the first kilometre of that particular training run didn't feel quite right. I didn't feel as relaxed and at ease as I usually did. At the two-kilometre mark, I began to feel discomfort in my left foot. I tried my best to ignore it, but five minutes later the dull throb had developed into a sharp, localised pain at the base of my third toe. It was as though a knife was digging into my foot, unlike any pain I had experienced in the past.

I was forced to stop. I rubbed over the bone, hoping the feeling would ease, and tried to start running again, but I couldn't. Come on, I told myself. Stop being soft. Push through the pain. But it was becoming more severe. As a physio I have always been fairly accurate in diagnosing my own injuries and I was pretty sure it was a stress fracture. Tears swelled in eyes as it dawned on me that I may have to withdraw from the marathon in Thailand. I hobbled home, feeling as though the world was caving in on me and my running days were over. I felt undeserving of any food so I went straight back to bed, praying I would wake up from this nightmare.

A bone scan the following day confirmed my fear. I had a stress fracture at the base of the third metatarsal (the third toe). I broke down when I saw the scan. I wouldn't be able to train for weeks, maybe months. I would lose my fitness. I would put on weight. I would have to further restrict my diet.

I rang Brent, unable to control my emotions. Tears flowed down my face, my hands were shaking and my voice trembled as I gave him the devastating news. I didn't want to go to Thailand any more. I couldn't get on the plane knowing that I was on my way to a five-star resort where I would be lazing by the pool with nothing to do but eat when I should have been on my way to a marathon. I would be overwhelmed with guilt the entire week. When I suggested to Brent that I cancel my flight, he told me to stop being ridiculous.

'But I can't come to Thailand knowing I should have been running a marathon. It's going to be all too much,' I cried.

'So you're telling me that the only reason you were coming to Thailand was for the marathon?' he asked. 'You weren't really coming to see me, were you?'

'Of course I was coming to see you,' I replied quickly. 'But it's just going to be harder to accept what has happened if I fly to Thailand and can't go north for the marathon.'

'Fine,' he said sternly. 'It's your choice.'

He hung up.

I looked at the phone in disbelief. It was the first time Brent had ever hung up on me. It dawned on me how selfish I had become and how twisted my priorities were. I wanted so badly to return to my former self. The girl who ran for fun, who didn't obsess over what she ate, who enjoyed socialising. Who was not delusional.

Next I rang my friend Anna, who was back in Melbourne and had suffered several injury setbacks herself, including a stress fracture. Anna and I studied together at university and from the day we met it felt as if we had known each other forever. We just clicked in a way I haven't felt with many other people. We finished each other's sentences, knew what the other was thinking, never had to explain anything. I knew she would understand the impact this injury was having on me.

'Oh Ness,' she said as soon as I broke the news to her. 'I'm so sorry. You know you will be back running in no time. Try not to let it get you down.'

She did her best to reassure me and it was comforting to hear her voice but I only talked to her about my stress fracture. Although Anna and I had always told each other everything, I couldn't bring myself to disclose the other, more serious issue that I was dealing with. The battle with the voice, my confusion, my compulsion, my obsession. I knew something had to change to save my health and my relationship with Brent, but how could I overcome my obstinate resistance to change? I felt withdrawn from the universe, controlled by the overpowering voice in my head, not quite knowing who I was anymore, what I wanted or who I had become. I was unable to find the bridge that would reconnect me to my former self and to others around me.

I gave it more thought and decided to go to Thailand. I knew I badly needed a holiday to give my body some rest and allow it to rejuvenate. And most importantly Brent and I needed to reignite the spark in our relationship.

I maintained a small sense of hope that my stress fracture would miraculously heal and I would be able to run the marathon. I packed my running gear and did not cancel my flight to Khon Kaen until twelve hours before my departure from the Sunshine Coast. I spoke to numerous sports doctors, seeking their opinions and advice, hoping that one of them would tell me it was possible to run a marathon with a stress fracture without suffering severe consequences. But the reality was that I would be in agony from the first step, I would most likely have to retire from the race, and it could progress to a full-blown fracture that would force me out of running for months. What would a professional athlete do in my situation? I asked myself. What would I tell my patients to do?

Under usual circumstances, I would have run for at least an hour before my flight, knowing I wouldn't have a chance to do any exercise for at least fifteen hours. (By the time I arrived in Bangkok, caught my connecting flight to Phuket and made my way to the hotel, it would be time for bed.) But I couldn't run and I had no access to a gym so I had no choice but to go without.

During the entire flight my mind was occupied with how many kilojoules I would have expended had I not been injured. At least six hundred. That's a lot of food I had to deprive my body of over the next twenty-four hours. We were served lunch and dinner on the plane but I only ate the salad and left the rest. I looked around me, watching everyone else devour their meals. Surely they hadn't been for a run that morning. How could they eat without feeling guilty?

The eight-hour flight gave me time to contemplate my diet and exercise plan during my week in Phuket. The resort had the most amazing array of delicacies, but I couldn't enjoy them without exercising every day. A cross-trainer in the gym would allow me to exercise without any impact on my foot. In addition to my daily sessions on the cross-trainer, I planned to do some interval sessions in the pool.

As the plane landed in Phuket I struggled to feel any sense of excitement. I couldn't wait to see Brent, but my enthusiasm was strongly overshadowed by disappointment and despair. I wondered what my priority in life was at this point – was it my relationship or my running? I couldn't admit the answer to anyone, not even myself. A few months of living on my own, with all my time and energy devoted to obsessing over running and my diet had left me oblivious to how self-centred I had become. I was ashamed at what had become of my life.

It was great to spend quality time with Brent but the week was overshadowed by my strong desire not to put on any weight. Despite daily one-hour sessions on the cross-trainer and sessions in the pool, I felt sluggish and limited my food intake at each meal. Brent hadn't said much about my training and eating habits, but during dinner one night, as we sat down at a restaurant on the beach, overlooking the ocean, he gazed intently at me.

'You look tired and you've lost more weight,' he began, his brow furrowed in concern. 'Why don't you just take a week off and rest your body?' In hindsight I know it would have taken him courage to say this out loud, aware that I would most likely shut him down as I had on previous occasions.

'I'm fine and my body doesn't need complete rest,' I replied abruptly, putting a small piece of fish into my mouth. 'I'm resting my foot, that's the main thing. And I haven't lost any more weight. I'm completely healthy, so don't tell me otherwise.' I looked down at my half-eaten plate of fish and vegetables – my staple meal when I eat at restaurants – ashamed, embarrassed, desperately wanting but unable to surrender.

'Are you eating enough?'

'What type of question is that?' I asked, my back prickling. 'Of course I am!' I continued to look at my plate, avoiding eye contact with him, fearing that he may be able to read my thoughts.

In truth, I couldn't reveal the extent of my obsession to him. How could I explain that my running and diet had absorbed me so extensively that it had become my only preoccupation? I could barely understand it myself, let alone admit that I was in vehement denial. So, with a flick of my head, I changed the subject and made it clear by avoiding his gaze that I didn't want the issue brought up again.

All Brent could do was shake his head. By the slow way he wordlessly moved it from side to side, I could see how frustrating it must have been for him. How challenging to continue to love me when each time he reached across the abyss, I shut him off so completely.

The morning of the Khon Kaen Marathon was difficult. The first thought that entered my mind when I woke was that I would have been at about the thirty-kilometre mark of the race and expended a lot of energy by now. Instead, I was lying in bed doing nothing. I felt the urge to do a gruelling three-hour session on the cross-trainer to relieve my frustration but, as it did on rare occasions, the sensible side of my mind took control and I realised how foolish that would be. One hour would be sufficient.

After a relaxing ten days, I returned to the Sunshine Coast still nursing my stress fracture. I felt more desolate than I had in a long time, alone in a state of bleak and dismal emptiness. My boyfriend was thousands of miles away; my family not much closer.

My running had been taken away from me and with it, the few running friends I had on the Sunshine Coast. In actual fact, they hadn't been taken from me, I'd left them. I didn't feel like being around other runners as most of our conversation revolved around running. Having few friends around and living alone with my boyfriend thousands of miles away had not worried me until now as I had been so focused on completing every training session, on how many kilometres I had run that week and how fast I had run them. But it was only when my running was taken from me that I realised how much it had taken over my life. Running was my life, and without it, I felt empty.

18 February 2006

I feel so lonely. I don't have anyone to confide in. Other than work friends, who I don't want to open up to, I have no-one to talk to about my obsession, my entangled mind, my strong desire to burn kilojoules. I don't even want to talk to Anna or Scott about it because I'm embarrassed. I don't want to disclose my mental state to anyone. I couldn't even speak to Brent about it when I was in Thailand. He tried to bring up the issue of my weight once but I completely shut him down. Don't know why. I'm ashamed, I guess. If I can't talk to my own boyfriend about it, then who? Where am I meant to turn to? Life sucks right now, I feel lost, alone, empty, my foot is still sore, I feel fat and lazy. And my running career might be over.

Each subsequent day became a little easier as I accepted that I had a runner's injury. With adequate rest, I could resume training soon. I thought of elite athletes whose injuries forced them out of important competitions – the Olympic Games, the AFL Grand Final, the World Championships. In comparison, my injury was insignificant. Running was not my profession. My life didn't depend on it and I was not in the media spotlight. I kept reminding myself that apart from my stress fracture, I was healthy – or so I thought – and what I was going through didn't compare to the suffering some people endure. Despite this, being forced out of running was devastating. It felt like the worst thing that could happen to me.

Boy, was I wrong.

9

Warning signs

A stress fracture is a frustrating injury. The bone scan can remain positive for up to a year after the initial injury, so there is no way to be sure you are ready to resume training. The only way to know is by trial and error. If you pass one session, that is, get through the session with no pain and pull up pain-free the following day, you gradually progress the time the following session. Four weeks after returning from Thailand I felt ready to test my foot out, so I planned my training sessions for the week and recorded the result of each. The first week looked like this:

> *Training session 1*
> *1-minute jog, 4-minute walk, repeat 5 five times*
> *No pain = PASS!*
>
> *Training session 2*
> *2-minute jog, 3-minute walk, repeat 5 times*
> *No pain = PASS!*
>
> *Training session 3*
> *3-minute jog, 2-minute walk, repeat 5 times*
> *No pain = PASS!*
>
> *Training session 4*
> *4-minute jog, 1-minute walk, repeat 5 times*
> *PAIN = FAIL*

I couldn't contain my emotions at the end of training session four as the tears ran wet tracks down my cheeks and evolved into uncontrollable sobs. I felt as though I would never get back to full training and my chances of running the Canberra Marathon in April were almost shattered.

I spoke to Scott, who advised me to take two more weeks off before testing my foot out again, so I continued to sweat it out on the cross-trainer. This time, instead of using the cross-trainer at the gym down the road, I hired one. That way, I could train whenever, and for as long as I liked without anyone giving me strange looks if I trained for over an hour.

I completed the same running program I had done for the past four weeks but on the cross-trainer instead. If an interval session was scheduled, I completed it on the cross-trainer. If I had a long run to complete, I would cross-train for the same amount of time. After nearly six weeks out from running, my frustration was immense. I was angry with my body for not healing more quickly. I felt the urge to punish it. To torture it. To push it to the brink.

My one-hour sessions became one hour and fifteen minutes and they soon evolved to one and a half hours. If I did one and a half hours one day, there was no reason I couldn't do it the next. Each session I pushed harder, my heart rate close to its maximum. My long session on Sundays began at two hours and quickly amounted to three hours. I did interval sessions three times per week, one more than what was in my running program.

I began to feel fatigued, sore, and there were mornings when I woke up with my heart racing – all a result of overtraining. My motivation levels were dropping, too, but still I pushed on, determined not to give in, in total denial of the harm I was inflicting on myself. I trained every morning at 6 am as missing a session would be to concede defeat. Each session my heart rate remained high as I pushed as hard as I could, a puddle of sweat forming on the floor underneath. There was no-one to tell me to stop. I finished sessions light-headed, my legs like jelly and struggling to support me as I hobbled off the machine – evidence I had completed a long, intense session. That I had pushed my body to the limit. To the edge. It was a sign of success. Of self-worth. Of control.

My obsession over kilojoules amplified; I was fearful that because I wasn't running, I would lose my marathon runner's body. You'll get fat. You'll lose your six pack. You'll be too heavy to run fast, droned the irrational voice inside me.

I no longer had 'treats' on Sundays and I continued to restrict my carbohydrate intake, satisfying myself with no more than a piece of fruit and a small tub of yogurt for breakfast. By restricting carbohydrates, especially after an intense workout, the glycogen stores are not replenished and over time, the tank becomes depleted. Can a car run without petrol? No. Can a car run with the wrong type of petrol? Yes, but not very well. When the body's glycogen stores deplete, the body turns to fat stores for energy – and when they are exhausted, muscle begins to break down. My body was still able to function, but far from its optimal efficiency.

Within a few weeks, my body fat had reduced to dangerous levels. I looked undernourished – my skin, sallow and taut, fell lifeless from my barely covered bones, my abdominals more prominent than ever – but my delusional mind saw otherwise. Although I ate an abundance of fruit and vegetables, there was never a day where I consumed enough to replenish what I had lost through exercising. My body was in constant kilojoule deprivation.

I am a health professional who helps people look after themselves, so my lack of introspection was shocking. I knew the facts well enough, I just chose to disregard them. I am now astounded that I continued to live in denial, overpowered by an irrational voice and blinded by a psychological disturbance that took me years to grasp and fully appreciate. I was so absorbed in punishing my body with gruelling sessions and monitoring my kilojoule intake that I failed to recognise my stress fracture was a warning sign – I never considered it was the result of overtraining or an indication that my body needed rest. I failed to see that this was the beginning of my body's rebellion.

I wasn't prepared to listen to anyone, either, ignoring orders from doctors, work colleagues and even my own patients to slow down and put weight on. I brushed off my parents' pleas to stop training so hard. So my body continued to throw dire consequences at me. And I continued to ignore them.

I don't know exactly when it happened because I had been on the birth control pill for a couple of years, but around the time of my stress fracture, my reproductive system began to shut down. My hormone levels dropped significantly and I stopped ovulating. I visited a doctor for a routine skin check and he told me upfront that I was too thin. He also asked me if I was menstruating regularly.

'My period is very regular,' was my reply. 'It comes at exactly the same time every month, to the hour.'

I was telling the truth. I knew exactly when my period was due each month and it never failed to show up on time. But what the doctor didn't ask was if I was on the pill, which was essentially giving me artificial periods. It wasn't my body doing the work but rather my regular cycles were the effect of a small tablet that I took every morning.

When another doctor asked me the same question and rightly asked me if I was on the pill, he suggested I stop taking it for a few months. I took his advice – and did not menstruate. It was no surprise considering I had the body fat of a lean child. I knew it was a result of my training and low body fat levels but I didn't care enough to do anything about it. I went back on the pill to protect my bones – long-term amenorrhoea (absent menstruation) can lead to osteoporosis – but it didn't set off any alarm bells that my lifestyle was detrimental to my health.

Did I eventually want children? Yes, but I would worry about that when the time came. I was still young, not yet married and I was a marathon runner. That was my identity. Being lean and running fast was far more important – I thought it would provide long-term happiness.

I finally resumed training four weeks after my initial trial. After two weeks of pain-free jog/walks, I felt ready for my first continuous run. It was the end of March, so the Canberra Marathon in mid-April was out of the question. Instead, I set my sights on the Gold Coast Marathon in July. My goal was still 2:45. Scott had no doubt that I could run this time, but I wasn't so sure.

I was surprised by how quickly I slipped back into my training schedule. I had not lost any cardiovascular fitness thanks to the workouts on the cross-trainer and within a month, I was running faster than before my stress fracture. One particular run erased any doubt over whether I could achieve my goal on the Gold Coast. It was a twenty-kilometre tempo run which I completed in 1:20 – exactly four minutes per kilometre. It had felt easy. I had felt light, strong and fast.

'Wow, look at you, you're tiny,' a friend from Melbourne
said as soon as she saw me. Clare and I hadn't seen each other in
over a year.

'You have zero body fat,' she exclaimed.

'Not true,' I replied defensively, misinterpreting her comment.
I was sure she was telling me I needed to put on weight and that
I mustn't be eating enough. I was sick of hearing it. I reassured
myself that I was perfectly healthy – fitter than anyone I knew and
running faster than ever before. My body must be in a healthy state.

Clare and I went out for dinner that night and I ordered my
standard restaurant meal – fish and vegetables.

'That's all you're eating?' she said to me when I ordered my
meal. 'No carbohydrates?'

'Nah, no need,' I replied. 'I don't usually eat carbs at night.'

Before she could respond I changed the topic, aware my
aberrant mind was doing the talking and I would have no case if
the conversation evolved into a friendly dispute. The meal I ordered
was healthy and nutritious, but for someone who had run twenty
kilometres that morning, which equated to over three thousand
kilojoules, it was far from adequate. I knew this, but I couldn't
bring myself to order anything more.

I was still hungry when I got home so I went straight to the
kitchen and devoured four non-fat yogurts and a bowl of cereal. I
had recently been giving in to my hunger pangs at night. I felt less
guilty doing this than if I indulged during the day. This pattern
of eating substantial amounts at night soon became habitual, and
I began consuming fewer and fewer kilojoules during the day to
'save' my kilojoules for the evening. I looked forward to sitting on
the couch at night with my feet up, knowing I had put as much as I

could into my day and that I had burnt as much energy as possible. I gave myself permission to indulge a little ... on healthy food. The voice in my head ensured that what I ate was low in kilojoules. If I did go over my quota, I had to run twice as far the following day.

During the first week of May I flew to Melbourne for Anna's wedding. Although our running events couldn't have been any more different, we both understood the discipline and training that was required to compete at a high level. We also both knew the importance of fuelling the body adequately for training. The only difference was that Anna practised it, I didn't. I have always admired her for her balance in life and I always will.

Anna's wedding was on a Saturday night near Wangaratta, a three-hour drive from Melbourne. A few of us drove up on the Friday to spend the day with her before the wedding. I didn't want to disrupt my training schedule, but I knew I wouldn't feel like doing my long run the morning after the wedding, so I did it the morning of the wedding. While everyone else had breakfast with Anna, I ran forty kilometres.

You may ask if I even thought about spending the special time with Anna instead of running. I'll answer by saying that sadly, no. I can't believe now that I couldn't even sacrifice one long run to have breakfast with my best friend the morning of her wedding. It is definitely something I look back on with regret.

A friend's boyfriend, Ashley, asked if he could join me for part of my run.

'Sure,' I said, aware that he was quite fit so would probably be comfortable running at my pace. 'But only if you keep up with me.'

I mapped out a ten-kilometre loop from our hotel, which I aimed to complete four times. I left bottles of water and electrolyte drinks in the car park of the hotel so I could rehydrate every forty minutes. Ashley joined me on my second loop, but struggled to keep up and only lasted five kilometres. I ran the last two loops on my own and completed the run just as everyone else was finishing breakfast.

They had kindly left some food for me but I ignored my body's cravings for the croissants, muffins and peanut butter sandwiches that were left out. Although I had just expended over eight thousand kilojoules – the equivalent of a loaf of bread – the manipulative voice inside my head told me not to overindulge. I looked around to see if anyone was watching as I carefully selected a piece of bread (no butter) and a piece of fruit. I didn't want anyone to witness my far-from-adequate recovery meal.

I also indulged in a small bun that I had bought from the bakery the day before. It had been my recovery meal after every long run for the past few weeks and was on my allowed list, so I consumed it guilt-free. A small bun was at least something, but I should have consumed five of them.

As an omniscient witness years on, I wonder why, oh why, didn't I ignore the voice, listen to my cravings and enjoy the food? I wouldn't have put on any weight. Those extra carbohydrates would only have made me healthier – and might have saved me from years of distress and despair that I was about to plunge into.

The wedding was great fun and for the first time in over a year, I even had a few drinks. I was tipsy after three drinks and the fourth drink pushed me one more step towards a state of drunkenness, but I was aware of my limits and switched to water. One interesting thing about being tipsy, which I think happens for many people, is that the little voice in your head which usually says, 'Don't eat this, it's bad for you. You'll need to exercise to burn this off just disappears.

I think I ate more chocolate cake than anyone else at the wedding. I enjoyed it so much, the chocolatey crumbs caking around my mouth and dropping from my fingers. I realised just how restricted my life had become and how little fun I had these days.

Only five years earlier, as a university student, I'd had no inhibitions, no limitations, no voice telling me what I could and couldn't put in my mouth. No compulsion to exercise to the extreme. I was a carefree student who loved to party. I was ten kilograms heavier, but I was happy. I desperately wanted to resurrect that person. The girl who never said no to dessert and who ate when she was hungry. The girl who didn't dread going out for dinner because she wouldn't know exactly what was in her food and how many kilojoules she was consuming. The girl who ran a few times per week to keep fit and felt so proud after completing a ten-kilometre run. The girl who loved team sports. And the girl who rested when she felt unwell and who didn't beat herself up about missing a training session. I wanted to be her again, but I didn't know where to find her.

I woke up the following morning with a splitting headache and a hangover, feeling like I had been run over by a truck. Why do people do this to themselves week after week? I thought. How did I used to do it? I dragged myself out of bed and drew open the curtains. The air was heavy with rain and the frost on the window made for a translucent white barrier.

I staggered across the room to where my running clothes were laid out. Come on, I tried to motivate myself. You'll feel great in an hour and you will have burnt lots of kilojoules. When the voice emerged, I knew I had no choice. You ate so much last night. Get out there and burn it all off.

Reluctantly, I got dressed. Leggings, two long-sleeved tops, a jacket, gloves, a beanie, socks and shoes, more layers than I had worn in a long time. I was ready to embrace the wet, freezing conditions. I ran fourteen kilometres and hated every second of it, my fingers so numb at the end that when I returned to my hotel room I struggled to turn the key to open the door.

Aside from Anna's wedding, May 2006 is a month I would rather forget. Brent returned to the Sunshine Coast from Thailand a week after the wedding – but two weeks later, we had a fight which resulted in him packing his bags and heading back to Melbourne.

A phone conversation the day before Brent was due to fly back from Thailand will remain firmly ingrained in my conscience and a sense of regret and shame will always remain with me. We hadn't seen each other for four months. I couldn't wait to see him, but his arrival coincided with my weekly long run. He was landing at 7 am on Sunday morning and I would only be halfway through. I couldn't break my run to go and meet him at the airport.

'Just take a taxi to my place and wait outside. You'll probably arrive at around 8 am and I shouldn't be much later than 8.30.'

'Are you serious?' Brent replied. 'We haven't seen each other in four months and you can't even cut your run a few kilometres short?'

'I can't,' I said quite matter-of-factly. 'It's part of my training program.'

'You've lost your mind,' Brent said bluntly. 'Running has taken over your life. And it's just about taken over us.'

'Maybe it has,' was all I could say, weakly.

I was on the verge of tears, totally aware of the truth in what he was saying. I wanted so badly to do something about it, but how? Once again I abruptly ended the conversation, wished him a good flight and said I would see him at my place when he arrived. His plane arrived on time, he caught a taxi to my place and yes, he waited outside for forty-five minutes before I returned home from my thirty-two-kilometre run.

30 May 2006

I can barely see what I'm writing, I'm so upset, tears are falling and leaving big wet patches all over the page. Brent and I have broken up. He has been here ten days and this morning we had a stupid fight over nothing and he threatened to leave me and fly back to Melbourne. I didn't believe him but I just got home from work and discovered he was serious. He's gone. So are his bags. No note or anything. This time I'm sure it's for good. The last ten days haven't been great. I did my best to spend more time with him, we went out more and I never complained about how tired I was but the spark's just disappeared. I know the tension has been building since last year and I know it's all my fault. My training, my irritable moods. I know I'm no fun to be around. I guess it all reached its climax and the argument was just the icing on the cake. I'm heartbroken. I feel empty. The pain of losing him is almost too much to bear, especially because I know I have only myself to blame. Myself and my obsession. Can things get any worse?

The week after Brent returned to Melbourne, I was struck down with yet another devastating blow – my second stress fracture. When my alarm sounded at 5.15 am I bounced out of bed, excited about being injury-free and ready for my long run. Why so early? Although I am blessed with olive skin that does not burn and tans easily – I only have to look at the sun to go a darker shade – I was aware of the damage the sun was doing and how important it was to minimise the hours spent training in broad daylight.

I had been running well in recent weeks and was feeling fit. A small pang of hunger turned my mind to the food I would be able to consume guilt-free that afternoon: a scroll, fruit, yogurt and cereal. I put on my training gear set up neatly on the floor beside my bed and downed two No-Doz tablets as I headed out the door. A hit of caffeine never hurts anyone at that time of morning and because I never drink coffee, the effect was tremendous. Within twenty minutes I felt like I was flying. As with all my long runs, I didn't eat anything beforehand. I could do without the kilojoules, and I preferred to save more for later.

It was approaching winter so the mornings were cool, but by the time the sun came up I could feel the rays warming my skin and my sweat rate increasing to dissipate the accumulating heat. At the one-kilometre mark, I felt a familiar pain in the middle of my right foot. Ignore it, I thought to myself. It will go away. I tried to convince myself it was my imagination, but there is only so much you can trick the mind into believing. I was feeling the exact pain I had felt three months earlier in my left foot.

Tears began to stream down my face, but I kept running. I couldn't believe this was happening. I was upset, mad, frustrated. I was so over it. I felt like punishing my body even more than

I had before, I wanted to force it tenaciously to the edge. I knew I was doing more damage and I could turn a six-week injury into a ten- or twelve-week injury, but I didn't care. Getting to the start line of a marathon seemed so distant and I wanted to give my body everything it deserved. It had let me down. Tears became sobs.

A group of young boys were ahead, staggering home from a night out. I bet they had more fun than I did last night, I thought. And they're not injured. I had flashbacks to my former self, to the fun-loving party girl of the past. Back then a stress fracture would have come as a welcome excuse not to exercise. It would have given me more time to hang out with friendsbut that realisation eluded me now.

I surrendered to the intense pain and limped home feeling very sorry for myself. I wished I could wake up from this nightmare. Maybe I should just become a couch potato, I thought. They don't get injured. They seem happy. Their bodies aren't physically tortured. My body was breaking down. It was crying out for help, pleading for rest.

My second stress fracture, which was in a different bone to the first, forced me out of running for six weeks. There would be no Gold Coast marathon this year, a huge disappointment since my parents were planning to join me and had already booked flights and accommodation.

I staggered to my bedroom, fell into bed and pulled the sheets over my head. I wanted to hide from the world and from everyone in it. If I couldn't run, what was the point? What else was there to do in my spare time? If I couldn't be a runner, who was I? My mind was spinning.

'Are you sure it's a stress fracture?' my coach, Scott, asked when

I gave him the news.

'Yes, no doubt,' I replied. I wasn't even going to bother having a bone scan I was so certain of it.

'You maintained your fitness with the last stress fracture, so I know you can do it again.'

'Yeah, I guess,' I said with no enthusiasm, my voice fading away.

What he didn't know was how much extra training I had done last time to punish my body. I knew I would do it all over again. I couldn't help it. I felt this strong urge that I couldn't resist. I had to. It was the only way I felt in control. I hired the cross-trainer and, ignoring my running program, jotted down my training schedule for the following six weeks:

Weekdays and Saturday mornings: 1 hour 30 minutes

Tuesdays and Thursdays: Interval session: 1 hour 30 minutes
Go hard every minute for 30 seconds
Get the heart rate up!

Sundays: 3 hours
* Important: must train for 3 hours to earn the right to indulge in usual Sunday treats.

The harsh words of the overbearing voice.

Based on the weeks that followed, I should also have written:

- *If you have nothing else to do in the evenings, cross-train for an extra 30–60 minutes. Why not burn extra kilojoules? The machine is just sitting there.*
- *If family or friends come to visit from Melbourne, do not let them disrupt your training schedule.*
- *If friends or family are due to leave on Sunday morning, make sure*

*you get up early enough so you have finished your session before you
say goodbye to them. If they are leaving very early in the morning,
it will have to be a quick goodbye while you are on the cross-
trainer.*

Aside from Sundays when my three-hour session allowed me a small
treat, my kilojoule count was not to exceed seven thousand per
day. Energy requirements (and kilojoules required) are calculated
on the basal metabolic rate (BMR). This is the amount of energy
needed for the body to function – for the heart to beat, for the
lungs to breathe in oxygen, for the kidneys, the brain, reproductive
system and other organs to function. For someone my size, the
recommended BMR is around five thousand kilojoules a day.

The body also requires energy in order to digest and break
down food, and then convert this food back into energy. This is
known as the thermic effect of food. Energy requirements also
vary depending on physical activity. For a sedentary person, this
is next to nothing. For the average person exercising for thirty to
sixty minutes at moderate intensity, it may be approximately two
thousand kilojoules. A ninety-minute session on a cross-trainer can
burn up to five thousand kilojoules depending on the person's body
size and sex. Considering the amount and the intensity at which I
was training, my body needed over ten thousand kilojoules. Did I
know this? Of course I did.

By the end of the first week I felt the urge to increase the
duration of my sessions. Another five minutes won't hurt. Go
harder. Longer. Get the heart rate up. Don't be soft. Burn, burn,
burn! So I trained for five minutes longer and another five minutes
the day after. Before long I was spending two hours on the

cross-trainer every day during the week and three hours on weekends. In the seclusion and comfort of my own living room, I would yell at the top of my lungs, driving myself to keep going, to ignore the lactic acid burning my legs and taking over my body. I pushed until my lungs were on fire and my legs were shaking, my heart pounding away, threatening to pop out of my chest. I thrived on the feeling. If I could do it one day, why couldn't I do it the next, and the next, and the next?

The morning of the Gold Coast Marathon I woke up at 8 am. I would be at about the thirty-six-kilometre mark now, I thought. I envisaged myself running along the main road of Southport, people cheering from the sidelines, the adrenaline pumping. I would be hurting all over but cherishing every minute. Instead I'm lying here like a fat slob.

I dragged myself out of bed and put on my bike pants and crop top. My clothes felt tighter. I looked in the mirror. My thighs were definitely bigger. My six-pack wasn't as prominent. I walked into the lounge room where the monstrous cross-trainer was waiting, ready to be pounded for the next two hours. Maybe I should try three hours, I thought. Approximately the time I would have been running on the Gold Coast. In retrospect, I realised what an absurdity this was – nothing but the reflection of an incoherent mind. But this delusion was only visible from the outside, to those around me. It was invisible to me.

After a long, intense session I stepped off the machine. I felt dizzy, my legs so fatigued they were shaking. I was dehydrated and thought I might faint. I loved this feeling. It was a sign I had taken my body to the edge.

A shower and a bowl of fruit and yogurt later, I sat down to study. I was studying a postgraduate certificate in nutrition by correspondence. Nutrition? you may ask. Yes, nutrition. I was learning how to fuel the body correctly and the nutrients required for optimal performance so that I could advise others. But I couldn't put it into practice myself.

My studies included sports nutrition, with a module on Anorexia Athletica and the Female Athlete Triad. I began to relate to what I was reading. These conditions resulted from low energy availability as a result of excessive exercise and disordered eating and were accompanied by amenorrhoea (absent periods). Other symptoms included fatigue, irritability, cold intolerance and anaemia. My iron levels were found to be low a few months earlier so I had begun taking iron supplements. And I could definitely relate to the other symptoms. I was also well aware that long term, this condition could lead to reduced bone density. I hadn't had mine tested – I was too scared. I desperately wanted to break my addiction, to exercise in moderation again and increase my food intake, but I just couldn't bring myself to do it. Any rational thoughts were drowned out by that powerful, internal voice.

After four weeks of cross-training, it was time for the test. I prepared myself for a very light, short jog on grass. My plan was to follow the same schedule as I had done earlier in the year when I had returned from my first stress fracture.

Training session 1
1-minute jog, 4-minute walk, repeat 5 times

Training session 2
2-minute jog, 3-minute walk, repeat 5 times

Training session 3
3-minute jog, 2-minute walk, repeat 5 times

Training session 4
4-minute jog, 1-minute walk, repeat 5 times

As I started my first session, I nervously anticipated sudden pain but I jogged the first minute with no pain. After a four-minute walk, the second minute of jogging was also pain-free. My third jog told a different story. After twenty seconds I felt it. A sharp, stabbing pain in the middle of my foot; a pain I couldn't ignore.

Training session 1: FAIL

I was distraught. Shattered. I wondered if I would I ever find myself at the start line of another marathon.

Little did I know that this setback would seem insignificant in comparison to the challenges that lay ahead.

I was so desperate to recover from my stress fracture and return to training that after talking to one of my patients, I decided to try alternative therapy. My patient's daughter had turned to acupuncture for several of her running injuries and although they were not comparable to mine, I thought it wouldn't hurt to try and she gave me the number of the person who treated her daughter.

'You're overtraining,' Jimmy, the acupuncturist said during my first consultation, after I explained my past history and a watered-down version of my current training load. 'You must slow down or it won't be long before you get sick. And I don't just mean a cold. Our bodies are not invincible. There is a limit as to how much they can endure. I used to think I was invincible too until the inevitable happened.'

Jimmy went on to tell me his story. He had been thirty years old, fit and in the prime of his mountaineering career. Training over one hundred kilometres per week and working full time, he collapsed one day and never fully recovered. He was diagnosed with chronic fatigue – a label used when nothing else can explain excessive fatigue and lethargy lasting for months. He had been forced to stop training for eighteen months and although he currently ran a few times per week, he knew he would never get back to the level he had been at previously.

I resented the fact that someone I didn't know thought he had the right to tell me what to do. Or rather, what not to do. But I can appreciate now that he was trying to help me, to prevent me from falling into the trap that had forced him out of the sport he loved. He wanted to prevent me from overtraining and failing to reach my full potential, too. But I wasn't prepared to listen to my parents, to Brent or to my doctors, so why would I listen to him? Why would I relinquish control of my body just because he had shared his story?

Towards the end of my first consultation, which was brief and only involved taking my pulse and looking at my tongue, he told me that my qi which refers to energy flow in traditional Chinese culture – was blocked and needed to be worked on. He explained that this was the cause of my recurrent stress fractures and that his treatment would prevent another one from occurring. Was I easily convinced? Yes. Gullible? Perhaps. I was so desperate that I was prepared to try anything.

After a few treatments I asked him whether I had made any progress and how many more sessions he thought I would need. At a hundred dollars a session, it was becoming expensive and I was getting frustrated by his unprofessional and abrupt bedside manner. He had spent a total of about twenty minutes with me over four consultations. The other one hundred and forty minutes I had spent lying on a bed with acupuncture needles inserted into various areas of my body.

'I can't say for sure. We will have to see how you progress,' he replied.

I couldn't monitor my own progress and felt threatened by this lack of control. His extremely vague response made me feel like I was wasting my time and money, so I didn't return. Most Chinese medicine practitioners will argue that I didn't give it enough time to see results, but my gut instinct was telling me that it wasn't going to work. And I didn't like the brief lecture I was given every time I saw him: 'Eat more. Exercise less. You're too lean. You're overtraining.'

10

Breaking point

One more month on the cross-trainer and it was time to test my foot out again. I started with a one-minute jog/four-minute walk session. I felt no pain and I pulled up well the following day. The subsequent sessions were also successful; a tremendous relief. Over the next few weeks I gradually built up my training. It felt great to get some routine back and within a couple of weeks, I felt as though I was making progress towards another personal-best time. I never thought I would say this, but I actually enjoyed my four-hundred-metre interval sessions and I was beginning to feel invincible again.

Brent and I had spoken a few times since his abrupt departure. Now he returned to the Sunshine Coast from Melbourne with the aim of rekindling our relationship. He stayed in his apartment, which was a very short distance from my place. I still loved Brent and there was not a day that went by when I did not think about him and wish we could make things work but at the same time something – I'm not quite sure what – was holding me back and telling me to move on. So I tried to resist seeing him but with very few friends on the Coast, I always said yes when he suggested we meet up for a walk or run along the beach.

This particular day the sun was shining, the sky as blue as I have ever seen it, the surf was out and children were everywhere – building sandcastles on the beach, riding their bikes and performing tricks on their skateboards. It depicted a postcard and provided the perfect backdrop for an afternoon run. Brent met me outside my place for a 'light', relatively slow twelve-kilometre run. We ran at a comfortable pace and I felt great early on, gliding through the air effortlessly, feeling the strong rays of sunshine tanning my skin. I remember thinking at that moment how much I loved running, wondering how I would ever live without it. Standing at six foot three inches, Brent is considerably taller than my modest five foot three inches and it felt as though for every step he took, I took two, but I was comfortable keeping up with him.

At the six-kilometre mark I began to feel strange. No words can describe exactly what I felt, but I knew something wasn't quite right. I had been cruising along easily but I was suddenly overcome with a wave of fatigue that I had never experienced before. I was forced to put in extreme effort to maintain my pace. I pushed on as I do during every run, determined to complete the distance we had set out to do. Anything less would be considered failure. At around the nine-kilometre mark I suddenly felt as if the world was spinning and my balance was off. With one kilometre to go, a terrifying sensation swept over me – I didn't know where my feet were.

Without warning, my legs developed a mind of their own, as if they were no longer connected to my body. What's going on? I thought. Why is this happening? I was frightened. My immediate thought was that I'd have to take more time off training, which would ultimately ruin any chance of running a 2:45 marathon that year.

I can't believe now that this was the first thought that entered my head. Was this truly the most important thing? What about the fact that I felt like I was going to fall over or my legs weren't connected to me? What about my health? Wasn't that more of a concern than simply running a marathon?

I managed to finish the twelve kilometres but collapsed to the ground at the end. A flood of tears streamed down my face. Brent did his best to console me, but couldn't. How could I explain what I was feeling right now? I stood up and took a few steps, but felt like I was on a boat. It was as though my body had been cut in half, disrupting the messages travelling from my brain to my legs. I was petrified.

I didn't say a word as I walked away from Brent, slowly making my way back home where I fell onto the couch, overwhelmed with exhaustion. I was more spent than after running a marathon. I felt dizzy and light-headed, distant to my surroundings. My brain was filled with fog, as if I was on a plane descending through the clouds and someone had opened the window.

I couldn't concentrate and went straight to bed, adamant I would wake up feeling completely normal, ready for my long run the following day. I had not missed a single session in the past two years. There were numerous sessions that I shouldn't have completed – who trains when they have the flu, or when their legs are heavy and sore from the previous day? Isn't that the body's way of saying it needs a rest? It was, but I hadn't listened. Each and every training session I had set myself a goal, whether it was to run at a particular pace or a specific distance or both, and I had used every ounce of willpower and strength to achieve it. I was sure tomorrow would be no different.

I woke in a sweat, my sheets damp and perspiration trickling down my back. My right foot felt numb. It's gone to sleep, I thought. It just needs to wake up. I tried to move it but realised the feeling in it was not going to return any time soon. Something neurological was definitely going on and my mind suddenly raced through every possible diagnosis. After about ten minutes the feeling in my foot returned and I got up to go to the toilet.

I nearly fell over, thinking I had missed a step down. I looked at the floor I was standing on. There was no step; it was flat. What is going on? I thought. My body was playing games with my mind. The body I had known so well over the past few years, that I had complete control over, was eluding me. My heart began racing. I glanced at my watch. It was 1 am. My alarm would be going off in four hours for my long run. Should I go to hospital? I wondered. No, don't be silly. You're overreacting. I crawled back into bed, threw the sheets over my head and eventually fell back to sleep.

I woke again two hours later hoping it had all been a bad dream. But the moment I lifted my head from the pillow I knew this was real. My head was spinning and trapped in a cloud of fog. The worst possible hangover cannot compare to what I felt, the dizziness and fogginess overwhelming. I took a step out of bed and experienced the same unnerving sensation as earlier – it felt like I was walking down stairs, but the floor was completely level. I began crying, petrified of what was happening to me. I felt so alone. It was 3 am but I called Brent, begging him to come over. I didn't need to say much. My voice told the story.

'You are not training tomorrow,' he said to me as soon as he arrived, his tone flat and firm. Words were not necessary. I knew I had no choice but to take my first day off training in over two years. My body was beginning to rebel. It was taking back control. Instead of running thirty-six kilometres the following morning, I went straight to the doctors. I desperately wanted Brent to accompany me but we were no longer a couple and I didn't want to rely on him all the time. So when he suggested he go home to have breakfast, I nodded my head, trying to hide the look of disappointment on my face.

'Are you going to be okay on your own?' he asked.

'Yes I'll be fine,' I replied. 'I'm sure it's just a virus or something. I'll be back running in no time.' I sounded anything but convincing; I didn't believe it myself.

'I'll give you a call later,' he said before kissing me on the cheek and heading out the front door. Butterflies entered my stomach as he kissed me, a feeling I hadn't felt in a long time.

The exhaustion was more profound than the day before but using every ounce of energy left in my body, I jumped on my bike and rode the fifteen hundred metres to the clinic. Despite the tremendous effort it took to do so, it was easier than it would have been to walk the distance.

I sat in the waiting room, my mind spinning, desperately wishing I was running along the beach. I could be burning so many kilojoules, I thought. Definitely no Sunday treats for me today. How ludicrous it seems now, how irresponsible that I was more consumed with burning kilojoules than focusing on my health.

My brain was still foggy and while my foot was no longer numb, my right leg just didn't feel right – I wasn't sure how I would explain these symptoms to the doctor without sounding like I had gone mad. When he asked me what had brought me to see him, I explained the events of the previous day and night. He listened intently, a small frown planted across his forehead. His look of concern did little to alleviate my anxiousness. He asked if I had ever felt similar symptoms before.

'No, never,' I replied.

'We'll conduct a series of blood tests, but it sounds like you have a virus,' he counselled.

A virus, that's it? I felt like yelling out. How can a measly virus explain my bizarre symptoms? I wasn't convinced. I had a feeling he had no idea what was going on and a virus was the safest explanation for now. I didn't say anything as he handed me a slip and directed me to the pathology room for my blood test – the first of a seemingly infinite number of investigations.

I went home and rested, but grew increasingly concerned as my symptoms worsened. The abrupt lack of control I had over my body was a frightening experience. It was as though it was deserting me, no longer wanting to be a part of me. I felt empty inside and more alone than ever before. It seemed like my body no longer wanted to be a part of me.

I thought back over the gruelling training regime I had put myself through over the past twelve months. I heard the echoes of voices warning me to slow down – parents, friends, coaches, medical professionals and other health experts. I had refused to listen and for so long my body had been pushed to the edge. Maybe, just maybe, I had pushed it too far.

11

Consequences

The next morning I was still feeling foggy and fatigued, but I dragged myself to work and treated more than ten patients throughout the day. Working as a physiotherapist is no office job; you can't just put your head on the table and close your eyes when you're feeling tired or unwell. You have to listen to people's problems, appear interested in what they're telling you, assess and treat them. It's physically and mentally demanding – and not ideal when all you feel like doing is crawling into bed.

Each consultation was a struggle. The most difficult part was listening to patients' problems and appearing sympathetic when I really wanted to say, 'At least you don't feel like your world is spinning and you're drunk.' But in the same way I approached every training session, I told myself I would get through the day no matter what.

My phone rang as I was packing my bags to go home. It was my doctor.

'Your blood tests show an elevation in Creatine Phosphokinase (CK). This is a cardiac enzyme and is an indicator of a possible heart attack. I need to admit you to the Intensive Care Unit immediately. An ambulance is on its way to take you to hospital.'

I was shocked. Surely I had misheard him. There couldn't be anything seriously wrong. Bad things happened to other people – definitely not to invincible athletes. I was sure I didn't need to go to hospital and definitely not by ambulance. This can't be happening, I thought. I have a marathon to run in a couple of months. I have ten training sessions to complete this week. I have sixteen patients booked in at work tomorrow.

I put the phone down and immediately called Brent.

'You have to come to work now,' I said, my voice trembling. 'I am being taken to hospital. I want you to come with me.'

He couldn't understand it. Just one hour earlier, he had called to see how I was and I'd told him everything was ok. I still felt foggy in the head and tired, but no worse than the day before. But I explained the call I had just received and told him he had ten minutes to get to my work as the ambulance wouldn't wait.

'I won't be able to get there in ten minutes,' he said. 'It takes longer than that to run.'

'Please, just take a cab,' I begged, before hanging up and burying my face in my hands.

He obviously sensed the urgency in my voice because nine minutes later, he ran through the door, a small bag slung over his shoulder. I broke down as I ran into his arms. Feeling his strong embrace and his familiar smell was comforting. I was suddenly struck with an immense sense of guilt at how much I had neglected him the past few months and despite how selfish I had been, how it was amazing that he continued to stand by me. I needed him more than ever right now and at that moment, being locked in his arms, I felt secure. It was the only place I wanted to be. It was where I was sure everything would be alright.

My memory of the ambulance ride is a blur. The only thing I remember is the nurse telling me that she had seen me running along the beach many times and was amazed at how fit I looked. She told me I had inspired her to keep exercising. Me? Inspiring? I thought. Here I am, lying in an ambulance. Really inspiring!

I was worried about my blood test results. Being told my results were comparable to someone who had recently experienced a heart attack felt like I had been handed a slow death sentence. I knew of a world-class triathlete who had been forced to retire from competition due to a heart condition. Was this the end for me too? I was only twenty-six years old and considered relatively young in the world of marathon running.

I didn't know exactly what was wrong, but I was well aware I had brought it on myself. I had only myself to blame. As I began to realise the enormity of my situation, a huge wave of regret washed over my body. I had trained harder and for longer than what my coach had told me to. I had ignored everyone else's advice to reduce my exercise and put on weight.

I felt sick thinking about the endless hours I had spent on the cross-trainer, testing my body to its absolute limit. I regretted my intense interval sessions that had other athletes looking on in disbelief. Many would be proud of such hard work and dedication, but at that moment, I felt nothing but shame. The words of a doctor I knew who also ran marathons echoed inside my head.

'Your long runs are supposed to be run at a low intensity,' he would tell me. 'You should be aiming for distance, not speed.'

I was convinced that I was doing the right thing by running all my long runs at race pace – I thought I knew better than him. I also regretted not listening to my stomach when it begged for food. And ignoring my body's pleas for rest. As I lay in the back of the ambulance with Brent by my side holding my hand, I bitterly regretted the last eighteen months of my life. Where had it all gone wrong? How had running, which was once an enjoyable, healthy hobby, become such a vehement obsession?

Nambour hospital is a large, public hospital. When I saw the number of people in the waiting area, I was grateful to be considered an emergency case and admitted straight to the Intensive Care Unit (ICU). Wheeled in on a wheelchair, I remember thinking: This is crazy. What am I doing here? I don't belong here. Hospitals are for sick people. I'm not sick. And I definitely don't need a wheelchair. I ran over one hundred and forty kilometres last week.

A nurse wheeled me towards an empty bed and helped me stand up. I wanted to tell her to let go, to let me stand on my own. I was not an invalid and I didn't want to be treated as though my days were numbered. But I thought better of it and smiled as she assisted me on to the bed. She informed me that a doctor would be with me shortly.

During my time working as a physiotherapist, walking from room to room, treating patient after patient, I never really stopped to think of the hospital experience from the patient's perspective. I certainly never imagined myself in their position. For a young, apparently healthy person, to suddenly end up in the ICU was daunting.

Brent stayed by my side, holding my hand. His warm, soft eyes gazed into mine, reassuring me he was there for me. 'Everything is going to be fine,' he repeated softly, optimistically. Words can't express how grateful I was, as I needed him more than ever. I couldn't stop thinking about how much he had supported me the past couple of years and how little time I had devoted to our relationship. He could so easily have chosen to walk away so many times.

I wished my parents were also there to comfort me, to tell me that I hadn't done any permanent damage and reassure me that everything would be alright, but I didn't want to call and tell them what I was going through until I knew everything was okay. I wouldn't be able to hide my anxiety, which would only cause them stress and make them feel helpless being so far away.

The nurse asked me to complete some hospital admission forms. As I wrote Brent's name as my next of kin, I realised with sadness that there was no-one else on the Sunshine Coast who could be called upon in this way. It reinforced the extent to which my training had taken over my life.

As I continued to fill in the form, a young doctor of no more than twenty-five approached me and introduced himself. He took down my history – a lot of which revolved around my gruelling exercise regime. He explained that he needed to run some more blood tests and a chest x-ray before a diagnosis could be made.

I don't remember much else of what he said. My thoughts were consumed with the alarming prospect of having done permanent damage to my heart. I couldn't help but think the worst. I lay in bed and gazed up at the ceiling as the doctor drew blood from me. I looked around at the cold, white walls. The sterility of the place did nothing to lift me from my solemn mood, from the fear of not knowing what lay ahead.

The doctor told me he would have the results within an hour. Following the blood test, I was taken by wheelchair to the radiology department for my x-ray. I was instructed to sit on a chair. As I stood up from the wheelchair I felt as though I was going to fall over, the ground uneven and my head spinning in a cloud of fog. I grabbed onto the chair to steady myself before sitting down. The procedure was quick, and I was wheeled back to the ICU. I lay in bed and waited for the results. Seconds felt like minutes and minutes like hours. The results could change my life. My dreams and aspirations could vanish in a few seconds.

Eventually the doctor entered the room. I felt anxiously ill, worse than before any race or important exam. Please, please, please, I thought to myself. Please let everything be okay.

He turned to me and said, 'The blood tests are normal.'

I breathed a huge sigh of relief and waited for a detailed explanation. There was none.

'How come the tests yesterday showed abnormally high levels of CK?' I asked.

'CK is often detected in the blood of endurance athletes,' he informed me. 'The amount that was found in your blood was minimal, but the doctor wanted to take every precaution. That is why he referred you here for more tests. With the amount of training you've been doing, it all makes sense.'

'What about my chest x-ray?' I asked him.

'That looks good, too. At this stage, we've found nothing wrong, so you will be discharged shortly.'

These words should have been music to my ears. I should have felt a sense of jubilation that I had not been diagnosed with a serious condition. I was healthy and could start training again soon. So why did I feel as though I had just been run over by a truck? Why was my head spinning and why did my legs feel as though I had just run an uphill marathon? I knew there was something wrong and I was desperate to know what. The stress and angst of the unknown only accentuated my symptoms. I so desperately wanted to stomp my feet and demand that more tests be done, but I knew there was no point. The doctor was already filling out the discharge papers.

Brent and I took a taxi back to my place. I tried to remain positive and reassure myself that nothing serious could be wrong if the tests had returned normal. Maybe it is all in my head, I thought. I knew how powerful the mind can be, and the enormous effect it can have on what manifests in the body.

As if reading my mind, Brent said, 'I'm sure you'll be fine. I think your body just needs some rest. Listen to it and give it what it needs. Why don't you have a month or two off training?'

'A whole month?' I exclaimed. 'No way. I'll have a few days off and I'm sure I'll be fine.'

As Brent often does when he disagrees with me, he opted not to reply. We both knew he was right, but I don't think he realised just how difficult it would be for me to rest. He was unaware of the daily battle I faced with the voice, with myself – and the dire consequences of time off from training. I heard the voice again: *You will lose your fitness and get fat.*

I rang my parents when I got home.

'Guess where I've just spent the last few hours?' I asked Mum.

At work, she probably thought. At the running track. Walking along the beach. Any scenario was more likely than in the intensive care unit of a hospital.

'Where?' she asked.

'In the Intensive Care Unit at Nambour hospital,' I replied.

There was silence at the other end of the phone. I could almost hear her heart sink. I imagined her jaw dropping open, her body freezing, the look of angst on her face as she scratched her hair nervously.

I blurted out, 'But I'm okay. There's nothing to worry about,' before she could think of a thousand and one reasons why I had been to hospital.

Stress is part of a mother's job description. My mother and father have always been there for my brother and I, always gone out of their way to support us, to comfort us; and they have told us endless times how precious we are to them. Whenever we were mildly sick growing up, my mother always said she'd prefer to be sick herself than watch us suffer. The last thing I wanted to do was make my parents worry, especially as there were over two thousand kilometres separating us. But it is not easy to lie to your own mother. I couldn't pretend everything was alright when it wasn't, so I explained the ordeal of the last thirty-six hours.

'What did they find?' she asked, concern creeping into her voice.

'Nothing,' I replied. 'Everything came back normal. There is absolutely nothing wrong with me. A good night's sleep is all I need.' I didn't sound convincing; I wasn't even convincing myself.

'I'm feeling a lot better now,' I assured her, 'just a bit tired'.

Positive thinking, I thought. I'll be back training in no time. My body is just asking for a short break.

'You're not going to work tomorrow are you?' my mother asked me.

'No, I'm not. My boss has given me the day off. I'll stay at home and rest.'

Rest. That nasty four-letter word that symbolised laziness had eluded my vocabulary for two years.

'Good,' was all my mother could say. 'Please, please look after yourself and don't do any running for the next week.'

'Promise,' I said reluctantly.

One whole week! It seemed impossible. My heart started racing at the thought of not running and stacking on the weight. I couldn't stand the thought of having the slightest bit of fat on me. I would have to buy new clothes. I wouldn't look like a marathon runner and everyone would start talking. What would I do on Sunday morning if I couldn't do my long run?

I said goodbye to my Mum, put down the phone and began to cry. I knew deep down that this wasn't just a small bout of fatigue. One good night's sleep was not going to make the dizziness, fogginess and unsteady feeling disappear.

4 August 2006

I slept thirteen hours last night! When I woke up this morning and saw that it was 10 am I couldn't believe it. Usually by that time I have run over twelve kilometres, expended twenty-five hundred kilojoules and treated four patients. It took every ounce of the meagre energy left within me to drag myself out of bed and onto the couch, where I stayed for most of the day, too exhausted to go anywhere, feeling too sorry for myself to see or speak to anyone and too depressed to convince myself that everything was going to be alright. I am scared to look in the mirror at the moment because of what stares straight back at me — a ghostly, white, gaunt face, the hours training under the Queensland sun not enough to disguise the pallor of my skin. My usually olive complexion is all but gone. It's such a shock. Every ounce of energy has been drained from my body and sleeping makes no difference. Today I walked from the couch to the kitchen every half an hour, a pang of hunger in the base of my stomach, but each time I found the will to turn around and return to the couch empty handed. I am struggling to put food into my mouth, knowing I am not burning many kilojoules. Why fill up the tank with fuel if I am not going to use it? You wouldn't fill a car with petrol if it was going to sit in the garage for a few weeks, or months, or years. I'm guaranteed to put on weight if I eat and don't exercise. To make things worse I have no idea when my body will allow me to exercise again — if ever.

I was back at work the following day, feeling a little better, but still not quite right. Colleagues and patients asked how I was feeling, but I knew I sounded insane when I described my symptoms, so I kept everything to myself. I greeted patients with the same smile and enthusiasm as always, provided the sympathy they expected and tried to be my usual energetic self. It was one of the hardest things I have ever had to do.

As I rode home from work each night that week tears rolled down my face, as a mix of anguish, anger and frustration bubbled over. Sure, I hadn't taken great care of my body over the past year. I was the first to admit that I had pushed it to the extreme, but did I really deserve to have to struggle through each day? To endure overwhelming exhaustion and constant dizziness? Did it warrant having my favourite pastime, my passion, taken from me?

Simple activities were a struggle: cooking, housework, showering. I was physically and psychologically drained. The daily phone calls to my parents became more frequent, up to three times a day.

'How are you feeling?' was always the first question Mum and Dad would ask me, growing increasingly concerned.

'I'm okay, just a bit tired,' was my usual response.

I did my best to sound positive, but sometimes I struggled to hide my emotions.

'I'm over it,' I cried one night. 'I'm so sick of feeling tired and dizzy. I feel drunk all the time. I know I have pushed my body too hard. I know I haven't looked after it, but I don't deserve this. Surely overtraining can't result in these horrible symptoms. I'm so scared it's something serious. What's wrong with me?'

I found myself asking this question many times over the next few years. My parents could easily have said, 'I told you so,' after warning me that I was pushing my body too hard, only to have me yell back, 'I'm fine! I'm running faster than I have ever run and I'm fitter than ever so please stop telling me I am doing too much!' But instead of pointing the finger at me, they tried to reassure me, telling me it was just a matter of time before my body would be strong and well again.

'Just please rest and look after yourself,' Mum would say.

'Yes, Mum,' I would reply. 'I promise.'

She'd heard me say this many times before, but this time I meant it   I had no choice.

The following week was a psychological rollercoaster that began with another doctor's appointment. This time I was begging for a referral for an MRI on my brain. An MRI, or magnetic resonance imaging, is an investigation to examine molecules that make up cells and tissues of the body. It is used to help diagnose various disorders and abnormalities.

I had done the most unadvisable thing that someone who has an unexplained medical condition could do: I had surfed the web. The wealth of information on the internet can be extremely useful, however medical information may be misleading or misinterpreted, often resulting in unnecessary worry and stress. Not knowing what was wrong with me was torture, so I desperately searched for possible diagnoses, and Mum and Dad were doing the same back in Melbourne.

When I typed in dizziness, unbalanced and fatigue on medical websites, the diagnoses that continually emerged hit me like a dagger through the heart: brain tumour and multiple sclerosis (MS). Could it really be? I thought. I was young, fit and healthy, a marathon runner in my prime. But at that moment I felt feeble, with barely enough strength to walk. I was scared of the unknown, petrified about my future. So one week since the onset of my symptoms, I returned to the doctor. He did not look surprised to see me.

'How are you feeling?' he asked when I sat down in front of him.

'Terrible,' was my reply. 'I'm getting worse and I'm really worried.'

'Have your symptoms changed?' he asked.

'The symptoms I had initially are persisting, and the last two days I have started feeling heaviness in my right foot and sharp shooting pain down my left leg,' I explained.

'Mmm, I think we need to run some more tests.'

'I need to have an MRI,' I blurted out impulsively. 'I think I might have a brain tumour.'

I was terrified of what the tests might reveal, but I needed to find out either way.

'Or I might have a neurological disease,' I added, as if our patient–practitioner roles had reversed.

He was still adamant that I had some sort of virus, but thankfully he understood that I wanted the MRI to put my mind at ease and agreed it would be a good idea to rule out anything serious. He gave me a referral to have an MRI and more blood tests. I rang the radiology clinic immediately to make an appointment. I would have to wait two days for the MRI, which meant three days – and three sleepless nights – before getting the results. Despite my fatigue and ongoing symptoms, I continued working, trying to erase the knowledge that I would soon know one way or another how serious my condition was.

Two evenings later I was in a taxi on the way to the radiology clinic when Mum called for the fourth time that day.

'How are you feeling?' she asked.

'A bit better,' I lied. 'Just resting at the moment. I'm still not running and don't worry, I don't plan to in the near future.'

Had I spoken the truth, I would have said, 'I'm feeling terrible. I'm actually on the way to the radiology clinic to have an MRI on my brain to rule out a brain tumour. I'm still not running because my body won't let me,' but Mum was already losing sleep over this ordeal. It wouldn't hurt her not knowing I was on my way to have an MRI. The taxi pulled up at Buderim Radiology Clinic and I made my way to reception.

'Please take a seat,' the receptionist said.

'Sure, thanks,' I replied.

I hadn't been able to stomach anything all day, sick from nervousness.

'Vanessa Smith,' I heard someone call. I looked up at a tall man of about thirty.

'Yes, that's me,' I said as I stood up and followed him down a narrow hallway and into a room filled with small machines.

'Have you had an MRI before?' he asked. His eyes were as blue as the ocean and he spoke with a soft, gentle voice. Hopefully he was used to patients being a bundle of nerves.

'No, I haven't,' I said.

'Okay, there's no need to worry,' he reassured me.

Easy for you to say, I thought.

'Please remove your clothing and put on this gown. The change room is just over there,' he said as he pointed to a small curtain in a corner of the room. 'Remove all your jewellery as we don't want any metal exposed.'

I did as I was told. It meant removing my bright red, moon-shaped earrings, my belly button ring which glistened in the sun while I was running, the silver ring with a turquoise stone on my middle finger that Brent had given me on our first anniversary, and a red and white necklace I bought during my last trip to Thailand. As I was put in a machine resembling a coffin, I really began to feel like I was unwell and belonged in a hospital. Lying on my back, I put on a pair of headphones to drown out the deafening noise of the machine – it was not dissimilar to a pneumatic drill.

I was informed that my head and neck would be submerged into a tunnel and I would be in complete darkness for approximately thirty minutes. He gave me a bell to ring if I needed to attract his attention. I nodded, indicating I understood and was ready to begin the scan.

Closing my eyes as the cover lowered, I let my mind wander off, allowing only good thoughts to enter my mind. I did my best to block out the noise, which was still loud even with the headphones on. I tried to visualise myself on a deserted island, lying on pure white sand, surrounded by crystal clear water with not a sound but the waves crashing and the birds chirping. I imagined I had just been for a relaxing swim and I could feel the strong rays of sun on my skin, injecting me with Vitamin D and giving my complexion a healthy glow.

Surprisingly, a smile spread across my face. I wasn't thinking about my next training session. I wasn't obsessing over the number of kilojoules I had consumed that day. Nor was I thinking about work or study. I was lying there, relaxed. I was at peace.

I was abruptly taken from my deserted island and brought back to reality when the lid of the coffin-like case was lifted and my headphones were removed. It took me a few minutes to adjust to the bright lights and realise where I was.

'Well done, it's all over,' the radiographer said. 'You may get dressed again. We will send the results to your doctor tomorrow.'

'Thanks,' I replied as stood up. It was going to be a long twenty-four hours.

'Everything appears normal,' the doctor announced as soon as I entered his consulting room and sat down on the large leather chair opposite him.

Those three words lifted what felt like a twenty-kilogram weight from my shoulders.

'Really?' I asked. 'Are you sure? They didn't find anything?'

'A small cyst has been found at the base of the brain, but it is of no clinical significance. Everything else appears normal,' he added.

I can't describe the sense of relief I felt initially, but the respite was short-lived as I realised there was still no explanation for my symptoms. The dizziness was constant, the fatigue had not subsided and I still felt drunk and unbalanced. The heaviness which had begun in right my foot was spreading up my leg and I still felt as if I had no control of it. The shooting pain in my left leg remained, too. I was relieved that the MRI was clear but I wouldn't be content until someone could explain what was going on or until my symptoms disappeared and I was reunited with my old body. The body that could run faster and for longer than most. The body that I had been so in control of. The body that had been invincible for so many years.

'What about my blood tests?' I asked, partly hoping something had been found which could explain my symptoms.

'The blood tests show a probable positive to a virus called Cox A. As with any virus, it takes time to get over it. You just need to go home and rest,' said the doctor.

I thanked him and walked out of the room. No neurological condition, no brain tumour and a probable virus. I wanted so badly to believe him, yet I was not convinced that we had reached the bottom of this.

When I got home I slumped on the couch and for about the fifth time in as many days, burst out crying. I was emotionally depleted, physically spent. I felt empty inside, all motivation and optimism drained from me. I had nothing to live for if I couldn't run. My family and friends were interstate. Brent was still only minutes away but I didn't want to become dependent on him. Besides, he didn't fully understand what I was going through. He couldn't comprehend the nasty symptoms that had seized my body and my paranoia over what was wrong. He didn't understand how distraught I was to have my greatest passion taken from me. Nor could he apprehend my fear of losing fitness and putting on weight and the guilt that swept over me when I put food in my mouth without exercising. No-one could.

I tried to enjoy the forced break from running and the sleep-ins, but my days were overshadowed by the stress of the unknown and the fear of getting fat. If I tell a patient they need time off exercise to recover from an injury, I assure them that it takes at least a couple of weeks to lose fitness. I also reassure them that in one or two weeks, you are unlikely to put on any noticeable weight unless fast food becomes the staple part of your diet.

Being in the position of patient, however, my mindset had reversed. Every time I put food in my mouth I literally felt it travel through my body and place itself on my hips. I was sure I would put on weight if I didn't reduce my food intake significantly. So I cut back on kilojoules at night, eating nothing but a salad for dinner and I forced myself out the door for a thirty-minute walk each morning, despite it being a tremendous struggle. I was as determined to complete the short distance as I had been to complete my long runs. Fighting an invisible external force made it far from enjoyable and I arrived at work each morning feeling as though I had run a marathon.

I woke up the following Sunday, two weeks since my initial visit to the doctor, feeling a little better. I spent the afternoon with Brent and was walking home when it suddenly occurred to me that I felt more energetic, more balanced. The world was no longer spinning and the brain fog had lifted. The heaviness in my right leg had also resolved and I felt like I was in control of it, as if the neural pathways between my brain and my leg muscles had been reconnected.

I cannot describe what it was like to feel normal again. Tears rolled down my cheeks but this time they were expressions of joy. I immediately rang Brent. My tone of voice said it all.

'I'm better!' I exclaimed before he had the chance to say

anything. 'I feel normal!'

'I want to give you a big hug right now!' he cried. 'I am so happy to hear you sound like this.'

The last two weeks had made me realise how much I took my health and running for granted and I have never appreciated good health as much as I did then. I was tempted to go for a run the following day, but having learnt a small lesson, I opted for a long walk instead. Despite still not running, the next few days were the happiest of my life. I felt renewed vitality. I loved walking and I loved work. I loved life. I also realised how much I had taken Brent's love and support for granted over the past couple of years. The fact that he had stood by me when he could have easily walked away reaffirmed his caring, loving nature.

After five days of feeling normal and void of fatigue, I couldn't resist the urge to run. I didn't consider it a training session – my aim wasn't to push my body as hard as I could or to complete the distance in a certain time. I was going out to have fun, to feel the sea breeze against my face and to do what I loved to do most. I left my running watch at home so there would be no pressure to run fast.

I only ran ten kilometres and I ran it slowly, but I have never enjoyed running as much as I did that day. My body was working again. All systems were operating and communicating as they should and my senses were in touch with the rest of my body. I was tempted to run longer, but for the second time that week, common sense prevailed and I decided ten kilometres would suffice. I did some stretches then sat on a rock and gazed out at the ocean, unable to wipe the smile from my face. I had been given a second chance. I heard footsteps approaching me from behind and turned around to see Brent.

'How are you feeling?' he asked me.

'I've never felt better,' I replied. 'And running has never felt so good!'

I could tell by the way his face relaxed, his smile came easily and the corners of his eyes softened, just how elated and relieved he was. He gave me a firm hug, the bristles of his face scraping my cheek, and told me how happy he was to see me with a renewed zest for life – and how difficult it had been to see me suffer.

12

Relapse!

It was 3 pm on a Monday afternoon when any hope of returning to training was shattered. It had been ten days since that glorious ten-kilometre run. I had run three more times since then and after speaking to Scott, who was doing his best to monitor my progress over the phone, I was contemplating resuming full training. It would mean following my strict training schedule, timing every run and putting pressure on myself, but setting challenges and aiming to achieve my goals was what I thrived on.

I was at work that afternoon waiting for a patient to arrive when the symptoms struck again. I started feeling tired and within half an hour I was swept away into my own hazy, foggy universe, distant from everyone and everything around me. As I tried to concentrate and focus on objects in front of me I began sweating as a wave of nausea swept over me. The fatigue intensified. I was forced to sit down, totally depleted of energy, the world spinning around me.

Fortunately, my patient failed to show up and I rescheduled my last three patients for the day. My boss told me to go home. The bike ride home was a tremendous struggle. My legs felt like they had turned to jelly, three kilometres felt like twenty, the slopes like massive hills. I couldn't believe what was happening. I can't do this again, I thought. I don't want to live like this. Surely I don't deserve this. The following day I was lying on my bed, too worried to sleep, too dizzy to read and too exhausted to get up. I didn't know what to do. It was difficult to comprehend how my life had changed so drastically. I didn't care if I never ran again as long as I could regain my health.

Invincible: the word haunted me. I felt a lump in my throat as I thought about the torture I had subjected my body to over the past twelve months and how I had ignored warning signs and discounted people telling me to slow down and put on weight.

As I lay on my bed and tried to visualise my body as strong and healthy, I imagined a water fountain inside of me. I turned it on to flush my body with clean, energised, rejuvenating water, killing all the nasty cells and replenishing it with fresh, new cells. This became a nightly ritual before going to sleep. The mind is a powerful thing and I so desperately wanted to have faith in my body's ability to heal itself. But with each passing day, with no sign of my symptoms dissipating or my energy returning, it was proving to be an immense challenge.

I mustered up the strength to walk to my computer, which was sitting on a table in the lounge. For about the tenth time in a month I went online searching for answers. The same conditions emerged again, which did nothing to calm my anxiety. I couldn't understand how overtraining and kilojoule deprivation could manifest as neurological symptoms. Chronic fatigue, yes, but what about the dizziness? My heavy leg and feeling unbalanced? I was convinced there was more going on. I had flashbacks to patients I had treated a few years earlier on the neurological ward of a hospital, terrified I was headed down the same path. My medical knowledge was not extensive, but I was haunted by what I did know.

'My symptoms have returned. I feel terrible. I don't know what's wrong with me.' I buried my head in my hands, embarrassed to be breaking down in front of the doctor but I couldn't keep my despair locked up any longer.

The doctor reassured me we would find an explanation soon. I told him I wanted to have an MRI done of my spine to check for potential nerve lesions, which may lead to a diagnosis of MS. Initially he was reluctant to refer me, but did so when he realised how concerned I was. He told me I would have to go to Brisbane, as the only MRI machine on the Sunshine Coast was out of order for at least another month.

Fortunately, I only had to wait three days for an appointment. How on earth will I get to Brisbane without a car? I wondered. The drive to Brisbane was over an hour, but I would work it out. I would pay for a taxi if I had to – peace of mind is priceless.

My mother sent me a text the next morning while I was at work. She wanted to know how I was feeling. My eyes stung, my eyelids felt like bricks. My entire body was hefty and burdensome, a huge effort to lug around.

Ready for bed, was my reply.

Despite feeling so unwell, I continued to work. I was contemplating how I would get to Brisbane and happened to mention it to one of my patients. Usually, it's about them: their relationship troubles, a confrontation they've had at the service station or the progress of their house renovations. I often find myself playing the role of psychologist as well as physiotherapist; an arduous task. But during this particular consultation, unintentionally, the conversation revolved around me. Aware of the challenging past few weeks (I had mentioned it to some patients) my patient asked how I was feeling. I explained how the demons had invaded my body again, this time with a greater vengeance than the first episode. I disclosed my fear of being plagued with an incurable neurological condition and mentioned my MRI appointment in Brisbane later that week.

'How will you get there?' he asked, aware that my only modes of transport were running and cycling.

'Not sure,' I replied. 'I guess I'll take a taxi. Maybe a bus. I'll work it out.'

'I'll drive you,' he offered, without the slightest hesitation. 'Let me know what time your appointment is and I'll pick you up from work. We'll allow an hour and a half to get there.'

His tone of voice indicated I had no choice in the matter. He was not asking me if I wanted a lift to Brisbane; he was telling me he would drive me there.

'No, no, you can't do that,' I said. 'It's too far. It'll take up too much of your time.'

What I really wanted to say was, Really? Oh, thank you. Thank you so much.

'What are you talking about?' he said. 'It's no hassle at all. You are not taking a taxi or a bus. I'll drive you and I'll wait for you while you have the scan.'

I argued a few more times, genuinely embarrassed at the offer, but he persisted until I accepted. I couldn't express my appreciation enough.

5 September 2006
I'm off to Brisbane tomorrow for another MRI. So over it. Going from doctor to doctor, having test after test is doing nothing to improve my health. It's really making me feel like a sick person. I'm ever so grateful to one of my patients for

driving me. I don't really know how I would have got there otherwise. I haven't told my parents about the scan nor have I told Brent. No point. My parents are too far away to do anything and I don't want Brent to feel obliged to accompany me. And I can't keep calling him and asking for his shoulder to cry on. I still love him and I want to spend every second with him but for some reason I am still resisting us getting back together. I'm trying to move on.

'These are headphones. They are connected to a radio to block out some of the noise. Here is a buzzer. Press the button if you need my assistance for any reason. The procedure will take approximately thirty minutes,' said the radiographer.

I knew the drill. This is what it feels like to be sick, I thought. Really sick.

Waiting, waiting, waiting. It was the longest two days of my life. What might they find? Was there a cure? Where would I be in five years? What would become of my life? The suspense was excruciating.

'Vanessa,' the doctor called.

I jumped up when I heard my name and headed to his consulting room. I was so nervous I hadn't been able to eat all morning. This could be the defining moment that I discovered my running career was over. Or that I was never going to fully recover – most neurological conditions are degenerative, with no cure. For years, my life was only of a high quality if I could run, but in recent weeks my focus on what was important had shifted dramatically. All I wanted was to be healthy. Please, doctor, tell me the results

are normal. Tell me I will be back to my old self soon. Promise me
I will learn to enjoy life again and I will appreciate everything and
everyone around me.

'How have you been feeling?' he asked me cautiously.

Was this his way of gradually breaking bad news to me?

'Not great. Still the same,' I replied.

He had my MRI report in front of him. As he read it, which
seemed to take forever, I studied his facial expression, trying to pre-
empt what he was about to tell me. My heart was beating fast and
a wave of nausea swept over me as concern spread across his face.
The wait was agonising. Come on, I thought. What is taking so
long? The word 'normal' doesn't take that long to read.

'It appears they did not do an MRI of your spine,' he said. 'They
have only done your brain. I requested for the spine to be scanned
but they have obviously misread my referral.'

'What?' I exclaimed. 'How can that be?'

I couldn't believe what I was hearing. I had gone all the way to
Brisbane and had embarrassingly accepted the generous offer of
my patient to drive me. And it had all been for nothing?

'Did they submerge your spine all the way into the machine?'
he asked me.

'No, they didn't. I did think it was a little strange but I didn't
say anything.'

'Well, at least this MRI confirms that there are no abnormalities
in your brain,' he reassured me.

This did nothing to ease the anger building inside. Combined
with my resentment towards my body and the indescribable anxiety
that had resulted in sleepless nights, I was ready to explode. I felt a
tremendous urge to scream and blame every single person around

me, to yell out at the top of my lungs that I did not deserve this, that life was unfair, that I hated being me right now. But somehow I remained calm. I waited for the doctor to talk, to explain the next plan of action.

'I will write you a referral to have an MRI on your spine, but you won't be able to have it done for three weeks. I have just been told that the machine in Brisbane is no longer working and the one on the Coast is not being fixed for three weeks.'

It took a lot of willpower to refrain from letting all my anguish and frustration out. I felt as if everything and everyone was against me.

'In the meantime, I will refer you to Dr Lucas, a rheumatologist who specialises in complex cases and undiagnosed conditions. He is very good and I'm sure he will have some answers for you.'

Great, I thought. I need a specialist, an expert in cases that no-one else has answers for. I took the referral and thanked the doctor. I went home, fell on the couch and howled uncontrollably, until eventually I fell into a deep sleep.

Getting out of bed each morning became more of a struggle, both physically and mentally. Sleeping was the only time when I didn't feel unwell and I wanted to remain in bed until my body returned to its normal, healthy state. My dreams were my only escape from reality – from my dismal, depressing life. Often I found myself running effortlessly under a crystal blue sky, feeling the wind in my face and smelling the salt-tipped ocean spray. I felt fit and strong and I loved life – until I woke up. I continued to speak to my parents daily, giving updates on my progress and how I was feeling. Brent and I also spoke most days but I didn't want to be a burden on him so I did my best to sound positive and assure him I was doing well on my own. I also spoke to my brother back in Melbourne more frequently, who was sounding more and more concerned.

The exhaustion remained, the dizziness and fogginess did not subside either, nor did the strange feeling in my right leg. I began to think I would feel this way for the rest of my life. The thought of running again was nothing but a distant dream. I struggled through work and put my studies on hold. Not only did I have to contend with the devastating symptoms and fatigue, but I was battling the voice in my head as well.

Fear of putting on weight consumed me. Because I couldn't exercise, I was forced to reduce my diet to fruit and vegetables. Anything more and a wave of guilt swept over me. More unusual symptoms appeared, each one adding to my stress and sending me back to Google for answers. My right hand felt as cold as ice, I had a strange sensation under my left foot that almost had me convinced I had stones in my shoe. My entire right leg felt heavy and my short-term memory was affected.

As hard as I tried to ignore the symptoms and urge them to go away, they weren't going anywhere. I thought I was going crazy. I couldn't erase the petrifying thought that one day I may not be able to walk. Where would I be in two years? Five years? Ten years? Would I still be searching for answers, my life consumed by endless medical tests? Would my condition be worse? Or would I have woken up from this dreadful nightmare and be living a normal life again?

I made an appointment with Dr Lucas the day I was given the referral. As is the case with most specialists, there was a two-month wait. The receptionist said she would put me on a priority list for an earlier appointment in the case of a cancellation. Thankfully, I received a call from her two weeks later to tell me she had an appointment the following day. So once again I found myself in a doctor's waiting room, trying to control my nerves by flicking through trashy magazines, terrified of what I might hear.

'Vanessa Smith.' I put down the magazine and followed Dr Lucas into his room.

He was a short, stocky man with a grey moustache. He nodded towards a chair opposite his desk.

'Now,' he said as he looked through my file. 'You have been suffering from several symptoms for a few weeks, is that correct?'

'Yes, it's been horrible,' I replied. 'I am living a nightmare. I just want to know what's wrong with me.'

'So you have had several blood tests and two MRI scans of your brain and it seems everything is normal,' he said, still scanning the papers in my file.

'Yes, that's right and that's the frustrating thing. How can they all be normal if I feel this way? I'm so over it.' I spoke louder than I had intended.

'I'm sorry,' I sobbed. 'I just don't understand why this is happening to me. I'm scared.'

Dr Lucas continued to read my notes, analysing every test result from the last few weeks. The probable virus, the normal MRI scans and the blood tests including the one which had detected a small amount of CK in my system. When I saw the look of confusion on his face, I knew the answer was not going to be simple.

'I see you were involved in intense training for a prolonged period of time. Your sex hormone levels are very low, as is often the case with endurance athletes. Also, a few of the tests for particular viruses have come back as inconclusive. I think we need to have these retested. I am also going to refer you to have your adrenal glands tested as you are displaying some symptoms of dysfunction, again a common side effect of overtraining.' Adrenal dysfunction – another condition to research online.

Overtraining. The word summed up the past eighteen months of my life. No-one had actually said it before. I had done my best to avoid it, and hearing it hit me hard. He might as well have pointed a finger at me and said: This is all your fault.

'Is adrenal dysfunction serious?' I asked.

'Adrenal dysfunction is very serious, but it is treatable. One of the symptoms is extreme fatigue. It is important to rule it out.'

'I'm sure what I have is neurological,' I said with certainty. 'I have all the symptoms.'

'Tell me what your exact symptoms are,' he said to me. 'And when they began.'

I explained every one of my symptoms. I mentioned the dizziness, the debilitating fatigue, the brain fog, feeling like my right leg was not connected to my body, feeling drunk and unsteady and feeling as though the ground was not flat. I talked about my heavy right leg, feeling like I had stones in my right shoe, the shooting pains down my left leg and my freezing cold right hand

Dr Lucas listened carefully, a look of grave concern across his face. I wondered if he thought it was all in my head. He noted everything down. He gazed at his notes then at my test results as though he was trying to piece together a puzzle. He glanced up at me, his gaze fixed for a few moments as if the answer to my illness was scrawled across my forehead in fine print. After what seemed like hours, he told me he didn't yet have an answer but he wrote me two referrals – one to get my adrenal glands tested and another to have Vitamin C and B12 injections, which he believed would help to restore my suppressed immune system.

He was adamant I would return to good health and he thought it was unlikely I had a degenerative neurological condition such as MS. His reasoning was that two MRIs had not shown any abnormalities and I was not suffering some of the symptoms that are commonly experienced in the early stages of the disease. I desperately wanted to believe him and erase any doubts in my mind, but it was so difficult to forget what I had read online – every patient suffers different symptoms, at different times, and sometimes a diagnosis can take up to five years.

I took the referrals and thanked him, forcing a smile as I walked out. I had treated pessimistic and ungrateful patients and I didn't want to be one of them. I made another appointment to see Dr Lucas two weeks later, by which time I would have had my adrenal test and started on the injections.

Once again, exhaustion made the ride home a struggle and I fell onto the couch as soon as I walked in the door. I didn't get up for over two hours. Two hours of not moving. Not exercising. Not burning any kilojoules. What has become of my life? I thought with horror. What have I become?

'Think of a time when you felt strong. When nothing could get in your way. When you felt invincible,' said Rebecca, a life coach in her mid to late forties. She had come to my work a few days earlier offering a free session. I needed all the help I could get, both physically and emotionally, so the opportunity to spend an hour with someone whose job is to inspire and encourage people to turn their lives around was timely. I certainly had a lot to turn around in my life.

I met Rebecca in the park and we had a casual chat about what I was going through and how I was dealing with it. She talked to me about the power of the mind and the body's ability to heal itself given the right environment. I didn't have to stretch my imagination to think of a time when I felt invincible. It had been less than twelve months since my memorable run at the Melbourne Marathon.

I would relive every minute of the race if I could, but the last two kilometres stand out the most. Despite excruciating pain in my legs I had felt strong and finished the race on the biggest high I had ever experienced. As I described the race to Rebecca and relived one of the best moments of my life, a wave of pride coupled with remorse and sadness swept over me. In one year I had gone from the greatest moment to the lowest point in my life.

'Every morning when you wake up, I want you to imagine you are running the last two kilometres of the Melbourne Marathon.' She spoke with a soft, warm tone and maintained eye contact with me as she spoke, indicating I had her undivided attention. 'You are fit, healthy and strong and you feel like nothing in the world can stop you. Lie in bed and visualise it, feel it, relive it. Over time it will become reality. If you want it to happen, you must believe it,' she enthused.

The vivacity I felt after my session with Rebecca was quickly dampened when another symptom emerged a couple of days later. I was walking down the stairs at work when my legs suddenly felt like jelly, as if they were going to give way. It was the same feeling I had experienced after my intense three-hour sessions on the cross-trainer. I grabbed the handrail to steady myself, waiting for the strength in my legs to return. I was able to continue down the stairs but I was terrified about what else my body had in store for me.

Over the next two weeks I had the adrenal test and a third MRI on my spinal cord to rule out the possibility of MS. The vitamin injections were painful. I could feel the ice-cold liquid travel through my veins during the entire twenty minutes. I was close to fainting each time. But the pain from the adrenal test was the most excruciating I have ever endured. I was injected with a hormone and instructed to lie down for thirty minutes, after which a blood sample was taken.

Sweat trickled down my back as the foreign substance was injected into my blood through a large needle. I felt nauseous, and again nearly fainted. After the test I was asked to wait for half an hour so the doctor could monitor my vital signs. When I was given permission to leave, I walked out of the surgery with not an ounce of energy left.

I returned to see Dr Lucas ten days after my initial visit, certain I would leave with a diagnosis and that my fate would be decided. I wanted an explanation not only for myself, but so that when people asked what was wrong, I could tell them. I preferred not to talk about my illness, but if people asked, I felt compelled to reply. Rather than explaining the details of what I was experiencing, I said I was dizzy and fatigued, two symptoms that most people can relate to.

The extent of my fatigue is difficult to comprehend unless you have experienced extreme fatigue yourself. 'Do you have chronic fatigue?' people would ask me.

'What is chronic fatigue?' I would reply, more abruptly than intended – I was frustrated at being asked this so often.

I know now that chronic fatigue syndrome (CFS) is a label

for persistent fatigue that lasts for more than six months, with no other medical explanation. Of course, anyone who is continuously tired for a long time is chronically fatigued, but the diagnosis fails to identify the cause of the fatigue. CFS didn't explain the other symptoms I was experiencing either, so my reply usually left people speechless and the subject was dropped.

When Dr Lucas told me my adrenal test and MRI had returned normal, I didn't quite know how to respond. I was relieved that MS had pretty much been ruled out and that my adrenals hadn't been completely destroyed, but there was still no explanation for my symptoms. The stress of not knowing was impacting on my life and my family's – my parents, after a long day at work, spent several hours on the internet each night searching for answers. And my brother's phone calls were becoming more frequent.

'What's the next step?' I asked Dr Lucas unenthusiastically.

I felt like this ordeal would never end. I had spent more time in medical clinics over the past month than during my twenty-six years of existence.

'I think it might be a good idea to see an immunologist. I notice from your history that you have travelled extensively through third-world countries. It is possible that you have contracted an illness which has remained dormant until now. When the immune system is placed under immense stress, dormant disease may surface,' he explained.

This was far from a definitive explanation, but it sounded reasonable as I had travelled through parts of Africa and South East Asia, including Kenya, Tanzania and Cambodia, and it gave me a small glimmer of hope. I sighed and agreed to follow his advice. Yet another medical appointment. More medical bills.

If only I could have seen then what is so clear to me now, I would not have spent thousands of dollars trying to get to the bottom of my illness. But I was blinded by an obsession, controlled by a voice in my head and in denial that by continuing to deprive my body of energy, I was not giving it the best chance to heal. So I continued to search far and wide for an answer to my symptoms. An answer that would point the finger elsewhere; never at me.

13

Still searching for answers

At the age of twenty-six I felt as though things couldn't get much worse. I had stopped working, my studies had come to a halt and I was feeling fatter by the day, despite still counting every kilojoule that entered my mouth and doing my best to limit them. I had no family or friends nearby except Brent. For a reason I was still unsure of, I continued to resist rekindling our relationship. I felt alone and detached from the world. I knew I had to do something to get my life back on track so when my parents suggested I come home to Melbourne, I didn't hesitate.

28 September 2006

I have decided to move back to Melbourne. I know I'm giving up life by the beach and exchanging sunny, mild winters for cold, rainy winter months in Melbourne, but I need to do something to escape this nightmare. This illness has made me realise that my family and friends are a lot more important than the sun and surf. I have neglected many of my friends the past couple of years. I hope they'll forgive me and let me back into their lives. And I need my family more than ever right now. I can't wait to give them all a big hug. I know they'll tell me everything is going to be alright. I know Brent will also move back to Melbourne but at least we'll both have family and friends around which will make it easier to be apart and to move on.

One week after making my decision, I mustered up all my energy to pack my belongings. I only had three suitcases to fill (two of which were full of running gear) and my bike, but it was the most exhausting physical work I had done in over a month. My colleagues took me out for dinner a few days before my departure and I was so tired I would have preferred to be in bed, but it was refreshing to go out and socialise for the first time in months.

As my flight took off bound for Melbourne, I experienced mixed emotions. I felt a sense of relief that I had taken the first step to regaining my life. I was excited about seeing my family and friends again, but there was a feeling of sadness at leaving the perfect weather and pristine beaches of the Coast. I felt a sense of regret that my lifestyle on the Coast had landed me in a state of ill health that I wasn't certain I could escape. There was a slight hint of fear, too, of not knowing what the next few weeks, months or years held for me. I landed in Melbourne and spotted my parents immediately. I ran into their arms and burst out crying. For a short moment I felt like everything was going to be alright.

Our first stop on the way home from the airport was to see a naturopath who I had seen six years earlier for asthma and hay fever. After three months of following his strict diet and taking herbal tablets, I had been free of any allergies for the first time since the age of three. His program had given me tremendous energy and my skin had never looked clearer. Through his assessments and various tests including urine analysis and an examination of the iris of the eye, he searches at a deeper level for the cause of symptoms than standard medical tests. If someone could help me right now, I was adamant it was him, so I made an appointment the moment

I decided to move back to Melbourne.

I entered his consultation room, bare aside from two couches and a coffee table. He sat down on his large leather armchair and gestured to my parents and I to take a seat opposite him. He looked at me with his small brown eyes, twirling the dark curls which framed his face.

'It's nice to see you again,' he began. 'How have you been?'

I knew I didn't have to tell him how tired and unwell I felt – my appearance made it obvious and was further confirmed by the difficulty I had answering his questions. My mum sat quietly by my side, her hands folded in her lap and my dad sat next to her, sitting back in his chair and looking just as nervous. I described my symptoms and I told him of my fear that I had a degenerative neurological disorder despite three MRI scans showing no abnormalities.

'That's great to hear,' he replied when I told him about the scans. 'Neurological conditions can be very difficult to treat.'

These words sent shivers down my spine. I hoped they would never return to haunt me. I told the naturopath about the detoxification program I had started a few days earlier. Through my vulnerability and desperation, I had been easily convinced by an online American company that their seven-day detox program would rid my body of the nasty chemicals and by-products that were making me sick. Testimonials from people who had miraculously been cured from illnesses after following the program had me easily convinced. If it could work for them, why couldn't it work for me?

The program included powdered drinks with vitamins and minerals and herbal tablets to detoxify the bowels. I researched the ingredients and found no evidence suggesting they could be harmful, so thought it was worth a try. The program banned the consumption of any food during the first two days – at least I wouldn't have to count kilojoules – after which I was allowed limited vegetables and grains. I was so hungry the first two days that by the third day, the allowed cabbage and cauliflower were heaven to my taste buds. When I told the naturopath about the program, he looked at me as if I had lost my mind.

'Do you honestly think you can detoxify your body in seven days?' he asked intently. 'That is absolute rubbish. We take years to make our bodies toxic. You cannot cleanse it so quickly. These programs are gimmicks.'

My desperation and vulnerability had made me gullible. Another five hundred dollars wasted.

'Stop the program and start eating normally. The last thing your body needs is to be deprived of energy. It needs energy to heal.'

I looked at my mother, who sat back in her chair for the first time, demonstrating a sense of relief about what she was hearing. I looked at her and she smiled faintly but didn't say anything, which I interpreted as 'I told you so'.

He is telling me I need to eat more and put on weight, I thought. He is just like everyone else. I took offence, but refrained from saying anything. His verdict was that my body was full of Candida, a yeast-like fungus that can cause infections in the body and was most likely manifesting as my symptoms. He said he would put me on a gradual detoxification program which included thirty herbal tablets per day and an eating plan that prohibited sugar, processed foods, foods with yeast and dairy. It did sound more reasonable and sustainable than the radical program I had put myself on. Because I had consumed very few carbohydrates and stayed away from sugar and fat for months I wouldn't have to change much. He said he wanted to see me in three months. As we drove home I was in far better spirits than I had been the past few days. I had been given a small glimmer of hope.

I have always been an independent person, but through my illness I was grateful to have my parents help me with the simple activities most people take for granted – cleaning, washing, cooking, grocery shopping. They all required tremendous effort and by lunchtime, I was drained of the minute amount of energy I woke with. I enjoyed spending quality time with my parents, although there were a few heated discussions around my weight and eating habits.

'You're too thin,' Mum said one night, a desperate tone in her voice. 'Please finish everything on your plate.'

As I looked down at the wholemeal pasta on my plate I wanted to yell straight back at her, to echo the words of the voice in my head: I haven't exercised. How can I eat if I just laze around all day being a big slob? I don't need to eat if I'm not burning anything. Please stop telling me to eat more! I hated fighting with Mum and I knew she was only trying to help so I told her I was full, kissed her good night and went to bed.

Three days after arriving in Melbourne was a day I wanted to eliminate from the calendar: the 2006 Melbourne Marathon. It was heartbreaking. Had I not been ill, I would have been competing, aiming to finish one or two places higher than twelve months earlier. It was a harsh reminder of how drastically my life had changed and that I had suddenly been forced out of running. I made every effort to stay well away from it, avoiding the news on television and not reading the papers for several days after.

When my dad mentioned the winning times after seeing the results in the paper the following day, I looked at him in disbelief and ran out of the room and into my bedroom, slamming the door behind me. I collapsed onto my bed, buried my head in my pillow and closed my eyes, trying to remove myself from this world and drift to a remote place, far away from this living nightmare. Of course my dad didn't intend to upset me and under usual circumstances I would not have reacted the way I did. But I didn't want to know about anyone who had run it, let alone who had won or what the winning time was. After several minutes, I composed myself and sat up. I looked up at the quotes on my wall that I had put up a few days before.

'Happier thoughts lead to … a happier, healthier body. Negative thoughts have been shown to seriously degrade the body and the functioning of the brain.' (Dr John Hagelin)

'You can change your life and you can heal yourself.' (Michael Bernard Beckwith)

'Remove physiological stress from the body and the body does what it is designed to do. It heals itself.' (Dr Ben Johnson).

The third quote carried the most relevance. There was no denying that I had tormented my body with immense physiological stress. My determination to control my body, my obsession with exercising to the extreme and my unwavering discipline had led me to where I was now. Since being forced to stop training, although not at my own will, I had removed this stress. Still, I continued to live in denial of the harm I was inflicting on my body in the form of kilojoule deprivation.

Every day I listened to the grumbles of my stomach as it begged for food. Every day I chose to ignore them, adamant not to give in.

I had studied nutrition and the knowledge that my body needed more was on the periphery of my understanding but wasn't enough for me to relinquish control. Staying thin and keeping my body fat low was more important. I knew I needed help, but I couldn't bring myself to admit it. I later came across a quote from Marie Cardinal, which perfectly captures the essence of what I was feeling. "I was ashamed of what was going on inside me, of this uproar, of this disorder, of this agitation; no-one should look, no-one should know, not even the doctor".

Not even me.

Six weeks after moving back to Melbourne I moved out of my parents' place and into an apartment with Roger. He was a friend from tennis who I had known for over ten years. We had been in touch sporadically since I moved to Townsville in 2003, but a surprise phone call just before my return to Melbourne proved to be good timing, as he was looking for a housemate.

Roger was four years older and a laid-back guy who I knew would be easy to live with. We moved into an apartment opposite the beach in Port Melbourne, a relatively affluent suburb not far from the centre of Melbourne. I knew it was going to be challenging having to do my own groceries, make my bed and cook dinner, but it was a step in the right direction. Although these chores took tremendous effort, I felt a sense of satisfaction and an increased level of independence.

Brent moved back to Melbourne two weeks after me. For the first month we saw each other a couple of times and spoke on the phone every few days. I still had strong feelings towards him and, other than my parents, he was the only person I felt comfortable talking to about my symptoms and how unwell I felt. Around Brent I didn't have to pretend everything was alright. I could be myself and his positive attitude was comforting. Our relationship was platonic, but he had indicated his desire to rekindle it. I still loved him and he gave me much-needed support, but I felt that I needed to sort myself out, find a balance in life and learn to love myself before I could commit to anyone else.

After nearly four months of not working, I had lost the motivation to get out of bed each morning. And since completing my postgraduate certificate in nutrition while staying with my parents, I had nothing to aim for, either. With each passing day, having achieved nothing and with no end to my debilitating symptoms in sight, I felt myself plunging into a sea of depression. Adamant not to surrender to this illness, I decided from that moment I would not let my symptoms stop me from doing anything, regardless of how unwell I felt. I was determined to do everything I used to do. Everything, that is, except run.

I started working at a physiotherapy clinic in the city. I had accepted the job just before leaving the Sunshine Coast, thinking I would be well within a couple of weeks. But during those first few weeks in Melbourne, driving to the city from my parents' place and treating patients would have been impossible. My new boss knew what I was going through and fortunately was extremely understanding and supportive. He told me to call him when I felt ready to start work and allowed me to choose my working hours.

I had more energy in the morning and was usually confined to bed by early afternoon, so I worked 9–12 Monday, Wednesday and Friday, allowing a day in between to recover from each shift. The three hours were arduous, but gave me a reason to get out of bed each morning. I knew I would get through no matter how difficult it was. I would feel a small sense of accomplishment as I made my way home and feel less guilty going to bed in the afternoon.

18 November 2006

I worked my first shift today. I'm so grateful that my boss has been understanding and has basically let me choose my shifts. I managed to get through but it was far from enjoyable. Listening to people complain about pain and trying to be sympathetic while I feel like this is difficult beyond belief. The commute to work is as much of a challenge as the work itself. I have cycled to work for ten years, regardless of the distance and the weather, but I just don't have the energy to ride the short distance into the city. Driving is out of the question – parking is a nightmare and atrociously expensive, and I don't have the energy or patience to be sitting in traffic. So the only option is public transport. There's a tram stop a short distance from our apartment and directly out the front of work so the commute couldn't be more straightforward. Except today it turned into a disaster. I took the wrong tram and ended up more than two kilometres from my apartment.

My old, healthy, energetic self would have been thrilled to walk home along the beach under the summer sun, smelling the fresh ocean air. But today, two kilometres felt like two hundred and I was so depleted of energy the whole experience was too much to bear. I broke down. I cried and I screamed and then I rang Brent, barely able to talk between sobs. I knew he couldn't come to rescue me because he was at work, but I needed comforting. As always, he remained positive and

reassured me everything would be okay. I was so distraught
that his optimism only infuriated me and I yelled at him
and asked him how he could possibly say that when I'm
feeling so dizzy, unbalanced and I feel like I'm about to fall
over with every step. How on earth could he say everything
is going to be okay? He didn't reply so I told him he didn't
get it and hung up. I feel so bad about it now. I cried and
cried as I dragged myself home. It felt like a tonne of bricks
were attached to me. That two-kilometre walk was the most
physically challenging I have ever endured. As soon as I
arrived home I fell into a heap on my bed and have only
just woken up, seventeen hours later, still dressed in my work
clothes. I just can't cope anymore. If I can't enjoy a simple
walk along the beach in the afternoon sun, what's the point?
How can everything be such an effort?

When I woke up that morning it took me a few seconds to realise
where I was. I mustered up the little strength I had to have a
shower, change into my pyjamas and clean my teeth. I went back
to bed where I stayed for the rest of the day. I needed as much rest
as possible before my three-hour shift the next day.

Despite my reluctance to get back together, when Brent told
me he wanted to take me out for my birthday, I agreed. I felt no
reason to celebrate, but I knew a night out would be nice. He came
to pick me up and when I opened the door, I felt like we were on a
first date again. He stood there holding an exquisite bunch of red
roses, beautifully accentuated with white lilies. As always, he looked
handsome, his striking ocean-blue eyes and his smile so gorgeous
I couldn't look away. He gave me a gentle kiss on the cheek and

told me I looked beautiful. I didn't feel it but it meant everything to me to hear it. As a true gentleman would, he opened the door for me as I got in and out of the car. He surprised me with dinner at a superb seafood restaurant in Port Melbourne overlooking the ocean. As we ate our prawns and scallops, he brought up the topic of us again.

'Have you thought about what you want between us?' he asked, gazing deeply into my eyes. His soft, gentle tone and deep voice were enough to melt my heart.

'Sort of,' I replied, not prepared for the question and wanting to avoid it. 'I just don't know what I want. I'm confused. All I know is I want to get better. I'm so sick of feeling like this. I'm really over it. You don't need me right now. Why would you want to get caught up with everything I'm going through? You deserve someone better.'

I'm sure it wasn't the reply Brent had been hoping for. I didn't want to dampen a beautiful evening, but I felt like I was suffocating, drowning, unable to pull myself from the depths of despair. This illness was consuming me and those close to me.

'What are you talking about?' he replied. 'I love you and want to be with you. I know you are going through the hardest time in your life right now. But I want to be there for you. I want to look after you and help you get better. You mean everything to me and it hurts me to see you so upset. We can get through it together.'

I felt a strong urge to jump into his arms. What more could I ask for in a guy? So many times over the past few months he could have pointed the finger right at me and said, 'This is all your fault. I told you to slow down and look after your body, but you didn't listen.' But not once did I hear these words.

'I just think it would be better if we went our separate ways. Especially for you. You know how selfish I have been the past few years. My running took over. I gave you nothing. And now I'm sick. Why on earth would you want to get back with me? Go and find yourself a girl who is healthy, someone you can actually have fun with.' I struggled to get the last sentence out, my lips quivering, the sense of remorse and anguish building again.

I couldn't stand the thought of him with someone else but I didn't know what I wanted. I was confused, my mind in disarray. I finally composed myself, apologised, and the topic was dropped. I tried to enjoy the rest of the night but by the time dessert came around I felt ready for bed. I didn't need to consume any more kilojoules either, so I said I was full. We asked for the bill and Brent walked me home, his arm over my shoulder. The walk home was a struggle, my energy levels totally depleted.

'Thanks for spoiling me tonight,' I said as we approached my apartment. Brent gave me a kiss on the cheek and then turned and walked towards his car. As he did so, tears ran down my cheek. I was in love with him and I needed him but for some reason I was fighting the urge for us to get back together. I felt confused, my mind entangled with mixed feelings and emotions. My sadness was further accentuated by the harsh reality that on my twenty-seventh birthday I had struggled to walk five hundred metres home from dinner. I could never have imagined this a few months earlier. I thought I would be training hard, running personal best times all over the world, feeling fitter than ever before – and loving my life.

During my second week at work and aware of what I was going through, my receptionist asked how I was feeling. I didn't want to sound like a hypochondriac and I knew complaining and focusing on feeling unwell didn't help, so I replied, 'I'm okay thanks. I'm getting better.'

She looked at me as if to say, 'I don't believe you.'

'You don't look well,' she replied. I was shocked at her response.

'Things aren't easy at the moment, but I'll get there. I just have to stay positive,' I said.

'I hope you don't mind, but I had a chat to my husband about you,' she said. 'He is a chiropractor who practices kinesiology and has helped many people recover from chronic illness. He has also worked with athletes who have overtrained. He would be happy to have a chat to you if you'd like to give him a call.'

Suddenly, our conversation took on a new meaning.

'Really?' I asked. 'I'd love to talk to him.'

'His name is Trevor. Here is his phone number.' She handed me a scrap piece of paper.

I was fed up with medical tests that revealed nothing and so far the supplements and diet the naturopath had prescribed weren't helping, so I was more than happy to try another alternative, natural approach to healing. I had no idea how a chiropractor could help me or what kinesiology involved, but I was keen to find out. Later that afternoon I gave Trevor a call and at the end of our half-hour conversation, I could see a patch of blue sky emerging from my dreary grey surroundings. I was given another reason to remain optimistic. I know a phone conversation doesn't reveal everything about a person's expertise, but I had a good feeling about this guy. He sounded good. Really good.

Two days later I was on my way to see Trevor. Mum accompanied me, as desperate as I was to get to the bottom of my illness. I arrived at Trevor's clinic spent, the forty-five-minute drive having zapped all energy from me even though Mum drove. I wondered how I would drive myself to future appointments. The waiting room was small but cosy. A video was playing which described the use of alternative, natural medicine to heal unknown, undiagnosed ailments without western medicine. It also portrayed a strong message regarding the power of the mind and its ability to heal the body.

'Medication treats the symptoms, not the cause,' the lady on the video explained. 'Unless you discover the root of the problem, you will never completely eliminate your symptoms; they will always be there ready to surface. With the right approach, in the right environment, provided you love and cherish your body, it can heal itself.'

Her subliminal message, to change my lifestyle and to start looking after my body, felt impossible. I just couldn't bring myself to eat more. I continued to listen and for a moment, there seemed to be no-one else in the room. I was sitting in a dark space, all noise blocked out. The lady was looking straight at me, talking directly to me, begging me to recognise, to disclose my confusion, my troubled mind, my delusion. She promised me that no-one was going to judge me for it. I listened intently and considered what she was saying. For the first time, I believed it. I wanted to obey her.

My eyes were glued to the screen and I was completely engaged in what the lady was saying when I heard my name. My surroundings returned and I was no longer alone as I looked up to see a young, slim man with a warm, friendly smile looking at me. He introduced himself and shook my hand and Mum's, too. Great bedside manner, I thought. One box ticked.

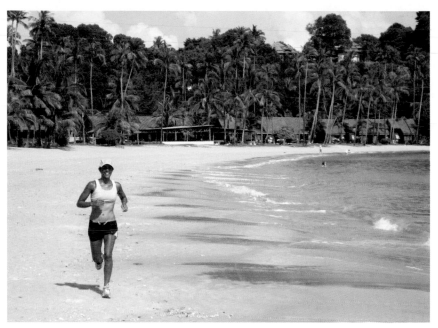

Running along the beach — what a way to start the day!

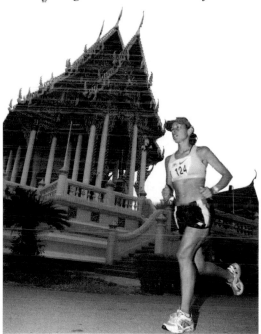

2004 Bangkok Marathon. Although my running mileage had increased quite significantly in recent months, I was at a healthy weight.

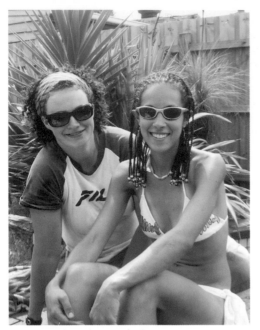

January 2005, a few weeks after my return from India – I was all skin and bones.

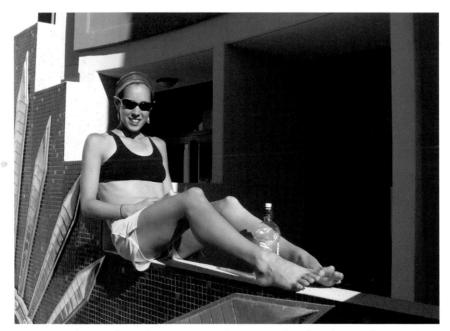

Living on the Sunshine Coast in 2005. I was very thin here but at the time I considered myself to be at my ideal weight.

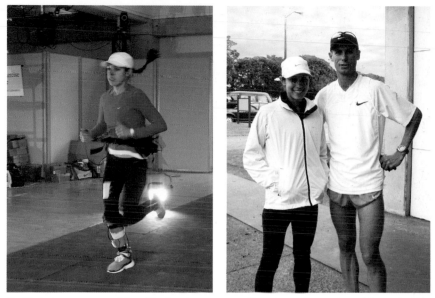

L: Training camp in New Zealand in 2005. Here I was having my biomechanics analysed to determine the most suitable shoe for me to train and race in.
R: Steve Moneghetti and I in New Zealand.

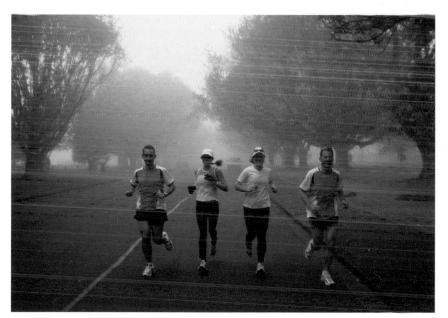

An early morning run in New Zealand with members of Team Nike. My gloves were a must!

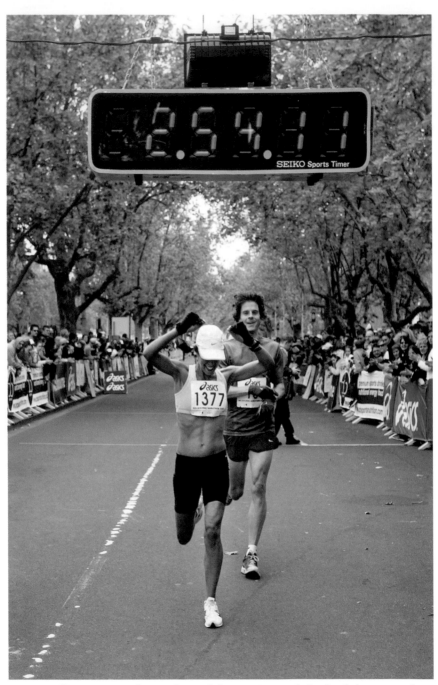

2005 Melbourne Marathon. What a feeling as I crossed the finish line in under 3 hours and in 3rd place.

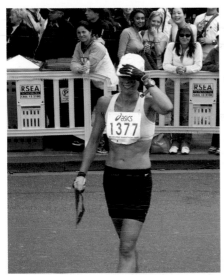

Exhilaration mixed with relief at the end of the Melbourne Marathon.

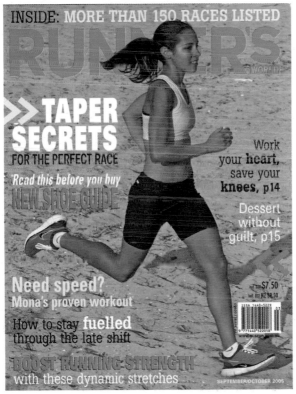

INSIDE: MORE THAN 150 RACES LISTED

RUNNER'S WORLD

>> **TAPER SECRETS** FOR THE PERFECT RACE

Read this before you buy NEW SHOE GUIDE

Work your **heart**, save your **knees**, p14

Dessert without guilt, p15

Need speed? Mona's proven workout

How to stay **fuelled** through the late shift

BOOST RUNNING STRENGTH with these dynamic stretches

\$7.50 (incl GST) NZ \$8.50

SEPTEMBER/OCTOBER 2005

2005 – The cover of Runner's World *Magazine. At first glance I look fit and healthy but a closer look at my shoulders reveals I'm far from it.*

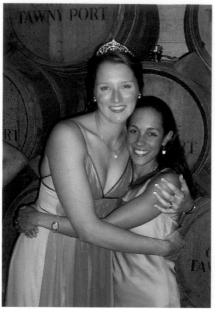

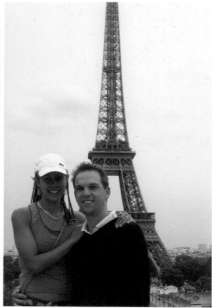

Anna and I on her wedding day in 2006.

One of our many visits to Paris, the most beautiful city in the world.

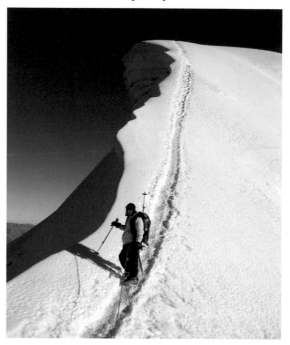

2008 - Trekking to 6000m in Peru in sub-zero temperatures was the most physically and mentally challenging experience of my life.

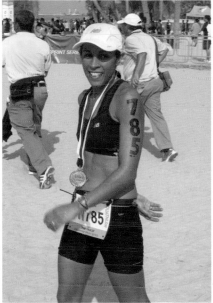

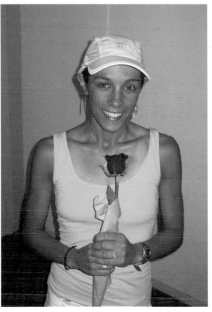

First place in the Singapore Triathlon.
I lived for these races.

In Singapore - although I was winning
races, I was clearly too thin.

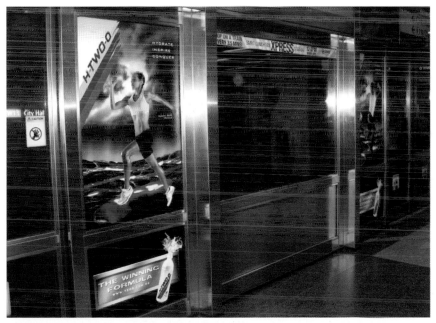

Within a year of living in Singapore I found myself on advertisements for a sports
drink in train stations, on trains and around universities.

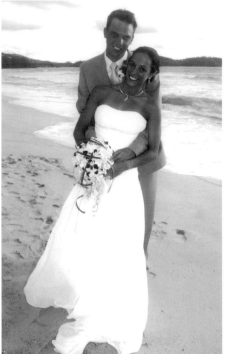

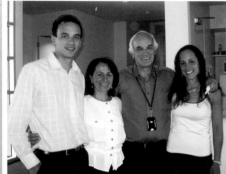

Left: 2010 – our magical wedding in Phuket, Thailand.

Below: My wonderful family – Mum, dad and my younger brother Steve.

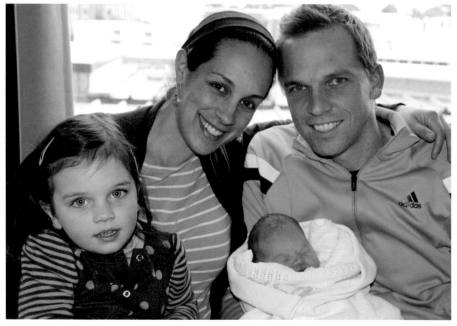

My husband and beautiful daughters, Mia and Madison

We followed him into a small, yellow consultation room with a treatment bed in the middle and two chairs to the side. It was brightly lit, which accentuated my brain fog. I sat down on the bed, my mother sat on one chair and Dr Trevor sat on the other. Immediately, I liked him. His soft gaze and gentle tone of voice made him very approachable and immediately I felt comfortable.

He asked me to explain what I had been experiencing, including the nature and onset of my symptoms. Because my symptoms were so unusual and fluctuated, and it seemed like I was in for a new surprise every week, I was using my diary more often to describe what I was feeling each day. The diary continued to provide me with an avenue to express my feelings and vent when I felt alone and detached from the world with no-one to turn to. It never judged me or thought I was imagining everything. No-one ever said upfront that it was in my head (except for an immunologist who believed depression was causing my symptoms and suggested I see a psychiatrist), but I know many people thought it. My diary listened to me and understood me in a way that no-one else could.

Trevor listened attentively as I described the events of the past few months. My mother sat in silence. I could feel her anxiety, aware this consultation would be a huge turning point for me. Each time I left a medical consultation without an answer, I was inconsolable for the rest of the day. I would either walk out of Dr Trevor's rooms distraught or elated. I described to him my symptoms, the results of my scans and the herbal tablets prescribed to me by my naturopath.

After half an hour of questioning, Trevor asked me to lie on the bed so he could perform his assessment. His techniques were unlike anything I had previously experienced. He pushed against parts of my body and asked me to resist. Some he did fast and some slow. He tapped on my forehead and pressed on my collarbone. He asked me to bend my right knee, turn my foot outwards and resist his force. He placed small test tubes by my side, one at a time, each time pushing against my hand and asking me to match his resistance. He asked me to stand on one leg, then repeat it with my eyes closed. I could only stand on my left leg for about three seconds; my right leg was even worse and it made me realise how much I was relying on my vision for balance. I was asked to adopt the tandem stance, one foot directly in front of the other and again with my eyes closed. He asked me to march on the spot and turn my head from side to side as I did so.

Following his commands was challenging and I found it difficult to focus on specific tasks. Trying to multitask and coordinate various movements of my head with my arms and legs was also trying. I felt uncoordinated and clumsy. I looked at Mum, the blank look on her face making it difficult to read her thoughts. I began to tire and I was tempted to ask Trevor what all these tests could possibly reveal, wondering if this would turn out to be another waste of time and money.

After twenty minutes, Trevor told me to sit back down. He scribbled some notes, paused for a moment and then turned to us.

'Do you want the good news or the bad news?' he asked me.

His voice carried a slight tone of optimism and I was prepared for the worst, so I said, 'Give me the bad news.'

'You are very sick,' was his reply. 'There is no doubt you have pushed your body to the absolute extreme, you have exhausted it more than what most would believe is humanly possible. Every system in your body has been challenged beyond its capabilities and it has told you enough is enough.'

My lips trembled as I worked hard to hold back the tears. I didn't need to be told that this was my fault.

'Is there any good news?' I asked, my voice quavering.

'The good news is that I will be able to help you. We will be able to get your health back on track, but it will take some time and work.'

'I'm prepared to do whatever it takes,' I said.

'I know you are,' he replied. 'I know what type of personality you are. You'll do anything to achieve a goal. That's what got you in this position in the first place.'

He was right. It was my Type A personality – ambitious, determined, high achieving and always wanting to squeeze more into one day than anyone else – that had resulted in me overtraining. Now I needed to use these traits to heal myself. If anyone can do this I can, I thought.

'Initially, I'll need to see you three times per week and as you improve, it will reduce to twice per week and then once per week. You will get there.' I started to relax. 'Before I begin treatment though, I need you to have two more tests. One is an x-ray of the spine, to ensure you have normal alignment and the other is a saliva test. The test will measure your levels of cortisol, a stress hormone and DHEA, oestrogen and progesterone, which are sex hormones. I have the test kit here. You will need to provide four samples of saliva at different times throughout the day and then drop them off to a pathology lab in the city.'

'What might the saliva test reveal?' Mum asked nervously.

'It may uncover any biochemical imbalances that can be the underlying cause of conditions such as adrenal fatigue, anxiety and chronic fatigue,' he replied. 'If they come back abnormal, then I will know what areas need to be worked on. I know you have had most of these hormones tested with blood tests, but saliva tests are more reliable indicators for these hormones. Can I ask you one more question?'

'Yes,' I replied anxiously. I had a feeling it was going to be about my eating habits.

'Have you had a natural period in the last few years?'

My head dropped in shame and embarrassment.

'I stopped taking the pill six months ago to see if I would get a period and I haven't had my period since.'

'That doesn't surprise me,' he replied. 'The reproductive system is affected in people exercising excessively and with very low body-fat levels. I suggest you start taking it again to protect your bones.'

I took a deep breath and forced myself not to take offence at his comment. He was just telling me how it was. He was trying to help me understand the necessity of making radical changes to my lifestyle. Maybe it was his professionalism, the way he explained things to me in a way that I could comprehend, that made me listen and accept these comments. Or maybe I was gradually untangling myself from the cobweb of denial that I had been caught up in for so long. I was finally trying to accept the help I knew I needed. But was it too late?

Trevor made it clear that I would need many sessions over a few months, but there was an aura about the man that gave me reason to trust him. He explained how one issue can potentially lead to another and can manifest as various uncommon symptoms that are unable to be explained by Western medicine. He had already discovered signs of fatigue in my body and possible causes of my symptoms, which he said he could reverse.

When he had finished talking, he asked us if we had any questions. Mum shook her head but there was one question I was itching to ask. It had been on my mind since the beginning of the consultation. In fact, it had been on mind for the past few months.

'Will I be able to run again?' I blurted out.

I am embarrassed now that this is the first question that came to mind. That running was still the most important thing to me. Trevor must have thought the question ludicrous considering my state of health. He looked at me for a moment without saying anything, an expression of sympathy on his face.

'Yes you will,' he replied with a gentle, soft tone. 'You will be able to run again.'

I started crying. Before I knew it, Mum had joined me. I was sure that comforting two emotional females was not in Trevor's job description, but he put his hand on my shoulder and reassured me that everything would be okay.

'Thanks,' I managed to say. 'Thanks so much. You have given me hope.'

The thought of running again excited me but still seemed so far away, so I tried to block it from my mind. I was encouraged, optimistic yet quietly cautious. I wanted to give him a big hug.

'You can thank me once you are feeling well again. For now, head to reception and make three appointments to see me next week. Then go and get your x-ray done. Don't forget to do your saliva test tomorrow and drop it to the pathology centre the next day.'

We thanked him again as we left the room and Mum put her arm around me as I wiped the tears from my face. Get yourself together, I thought. This is ridiculous.

From that moment I stopped taking the herbal tablets prescribed to me by the naturopath and decided not to return to see him. Instead, I focused all my energy towards Trevor's treatment. I saw Trevor ten times during the weeks leading up to Christmas, and by the new year I was still seeing him twice a week. The saliva tests had confirmed his predictions: my cortisol levels were extremely high. Trevor explained that cortisol is a hormone secreted by the adrenal glands in response to stress or exercise. When you exercise, cortisol levels increase, then they decrease once you stop exercising. Because I had continuously stressed my body without giving it sufficient (or any) time to recover, my cortisol levels had remained elevated. As a result, my levels had risen to twenty times what was considered normal.

Cortisol can have nasty effects on all parts of the body, including the brain. Trevor explained that my excessively high levels may have affected my nervous system, which explained my neurological symptoms. The cortisol was also causing fatigue. For the first time since the onset of my symptoms, I felt like the puzzle that was my illness was slowly being pieced together. I was beginning to appreciate how the different parts intertwined.

Trevor's treatment involved similar techniques to his assessment. I had to try and match his resistance, he did some tapping on particular points on my body, he pushed down on other areas, I was asked to hum, to count to five and to march on the spot. The sessions lasted approximately fifteen minutes, after which he would tell me I was doing well. I didn't quite know what he meant because I hadn't noticed any improvement in my symptoms and I felt useless lying on the treatment bed following his orders. But I forced myself to believe him.

He put me on a similar diet to the one I was following from the naturopath, prohibiting processed foods and sugar. I hadn't exercised in over three months, and continued to limit my kilojoule intake, so his diet was a blessing. He also prohibited any nightshade vegetables – eggplant, red capsicum, chilli. I didn't ask why, I just obeyed. I was tired of trying to analyse everything I was told so I decided to take a different approach – to trust, listen and obey the experts.

One week after my first treatment session with Trevor I saw a neurologist. I had booked the appointment a couple of months earlier as even though three MRIs had returned clear, my neurological symptoms had increased in severity. Still struggling to accept that my symptoms were self-inflicted, my parents and I thought it would be worth seeing a specialist. I was reluctant to go, adamant that Trevor had me on the right track, but I had waited over two months and I figured it couldn't hurt to obtain a specialist's opinion.

I had been sitting in the waiting room for no longer than five minutes when a tall, slim man with short grey hair appeared. He introduced himself as Dr Faraday and as I entered his consulting room, he gestured to a large chair in front of his desk.

'What can I do for you today?' he asked from behind his desk.

I began to explain the occurrences of the past couple of months and passed him my MRI reports.

'That's great that they have returned normal,' he said.

He conducted his physical assessment and then sat back down in his chair.

'At this stage, I don't think it is necessary to conduct any more tests. See how you go over the next six months and come back and see me if your symptoms haven't improved by the middle of next year.'

I told him about Trevor and his treatment.

'I guess it can't hurt, but don't expect any miracles.' His scepticism, portraying nothing but ignorance towards natural therapies, infuriated me. I barely looked at him as I thanked him and stood up to leave the room. Another waste of time and money, I thought.

I felt no reason to celebrate New Year's Eve. I knew I would be ready for bed by 6 pm and everyone would be consuming vast amounts of alcohol, which was on Trevor's prohibited list. After four weeks following his diet I didn't want to jeopardise my recovery in one night. But when friends insisted that a night out would do me good and pointed out that I had not gone out with them since moving back from the Sunshine Coast, I gave it another thought. They had a valid point – since moving back to Melbourne, aside from the occasional dinner, I had not been out. Socialising was the last thing I felt like doing. But it was New Year's Eve, after all, so I decided to try and have a fun night out with friends.

The night began with a barbeque at a friend's place. I brought my own piece of fish as I knew the hamburgers and sausages that are the staple of any Australian barbeque would be packed with kilojoules. In hindsight, how ridiculous it was for me to bring my own piece of fish, how embarrassing. I cringe when I consider that my actions were exposing the very thing I wanted hidden. I think now how obvious it must have been that my eating was disordered, but at the time, caught up in it all, I was so unaware of others' perceptions.

After dinner we proceeded to a bar in St Kilda, contending with thousands of other people. It was a scorching hot evening and sweat ran down the back of my legs. Inside the bar it was even more stifling. The suffocating room reminded me why I had not been out to a bar or nightclub in over five years. Staying at home on a Saturday night, going to bed early and getting up for my long run was far more appealing than standing in a room packed with hundreds of sweaty, intoxicated stumbling people, strong body odour hanging in the air and the occasional sleazy hand running along your backside.

By 10 pm I was ready to go home, but I had promised myself I would make it until midnight. I was going to at least try and have fun. The night did get better when a good-looking guy, tall, muscular with short dark hair and bronzed skin, asked me if I wanted a drink.

What was I supposed to say? 'Ah, I'll just have a fruit juice as I'm seeing a kinesiologist who has given me strict orders not to drink. Just a small glass, too, as I'm obsessed with counting kilojoules.' The guy would think I was a lunatic.

'Sure,' I said.

Call it peer pressure or some other type of pressure, but after four weeks of religiously adhering to Trevor's diet, I drank a glass of vodka mixed with raspberry soda. A battle between two voices went on inside my head.

One voice told me I was consuming empty kilojoules that I hadn't expended and that I would be set back another couple of months on my road to recovery. The other voice told me to relax and have fun. It was New Year's Eve and it was okay to have one or two drinks. I tried to believe the latter. The guy who bought me the drink was on holiday from the US. He complimented me on how I looked and asked me why I didn't have a boyfriend. What was I meant to say? 'Because I've been so obsessed with exercise the past few years no guy would want to go out with me when I prefer to run twenty kilometres than spend time with him.' Alternatively, 'I'm actually really sick and messed up at the moment and I resent myself for the torture I have inflicted on my body so no-one could possibly love me when I don't even love myself.'

Instead, I didn't say anything. I just shrugged and fired the same question back. We must have been chatting for over an hour because we were still in deep conversation when the countdown to the new year began.

'Ten, nine, eight, seven, six, five, four, three, two, one … happy new year!'

By midnight, nearly everyone was drunk and there were hugs and kisses all round. Fun if you're also tipsy, but repulsive if you're sober. Just after midnight my friends told me they were ready to leave and asked me if I wanted to join them.

'Already?' I asked. I could have continued our conversation into the early hours of the morning but I wanted to stay with my friends. The guy gave me his phone number and told me he would love to see me again while he was still in Melbourne.

'Give me a call sometime this week,' he said as he gave me a kiss on the cheek.

'Will do,' I said. We left and headed to a bar down the road. As is so often the case with people you meet out, I never called him.

By 2 am I was beginning to tire – 2 am! I couldn't believe I had lasted so long. It was the latest I had stayed up for months. My friends were catching a taxi home but they lived in the opposite direction so I told them I would get a separate one. The queue for taxis was atrociously long – at least a forty-five-minute wait and I knew I could just about walk home in that time (well, my healthy body could have anyway).

I decided to start walking. I would hail a cab when the fatigue hit. My one vodka and soda had quickly become three and I was feeling a little dazed. It was a nice feeling and for the first time since my illness, I felt almost invincible. If I'd had my running shoes, I'm sure I would have tried to run. Instead I removed my high heels from my aching feet and began the five-kilometre walk home.

Just as I approached every training session, I set myself a small goal. My aim was to walk two kilometres before hailing a taxi. I reached the two-kilometre mark and felt okay, so I told myself I could make it to three kilometres. Thirty minutes later I was still walking and my apartment was within sight. There's no point getting a taxi now, I thought. Before I knew it I was home. It was past 3 am. I had walked five kilometres. It felt like a major milestone in my recovery.

14

2007 Despair

The 2007 Australian Open will always remain etched in my memory, but for all the wrong reasons. The interesting people I met and the great matches that were played are overshadowed by memories of struggling to walk around the grounds, feeling as though I had been injected with poison. I felt so fatigued and feeble, the jelly-like feeling in my legs so debilitating that it took a tremendous effort to make it up fifteen stairs. I watched a friend play his doubles match but was too tired to stay until the end. And just when I thought I couldn't possibly be hit with more symptoms, I was wrong. As I made my way to a food stand to buy a drink it suddenly felt like someone was stretching the skin on the back of my legs. As if I was wearing leggings three sizes too small that were constricting my legs. What else did my body have in store for me?

To rub further salt into my emotional wounds, I had agreed to meet Jack, a friend who used to join me on my long runs on the Sunshine Coast. We had covered endless miles together that allowed for much conversation. I hadn't seen him since leaving the Coast four months earlier. I had never explained my abrupt departure or why I was forced to suddenly stop running. He probably thought I had a common runner's injury that would just require a few weeks of rest, so the first thing he asked was how my running was going.

'I'm struggling to walk around the grounds at the moment,' I admitted.

To the naked eye there was nothing wrong with me, so his

question was valid, but it was clear from my abrupt response that I didn't want to talk about it.

'How is your running going?' I forced myself to ask.

He told me he had a knee injury and hadn't been able to train for seven weeks. A few months ago I would have felt immense sympathy for him. Such an injury seemed like the end of the world, the worst possible thing that could happen to a runner. But right now a knee injury could not have appeared more insignificant. Jack called me a few times after that day but I did not return his calls. I didn't want any reminders of my time as a runner. I haven't spoken to him since, nor have I been in touch with anyone else I used to run with on the Coast. Losing these friendships is just one regret I have from my troubled years.

27 January 2007

Bad day. Very tired. Legs have felt like jelly all day. I had an appointment with Trevor this morning. He said I have improved but apart from a slight increase in my energy levels, I don't feel it.

I was watching someone run along the beach this afternoon with envy. Running just looks like such an effort. I don't think I will ever be able to run again. This time last year I was hit with my first stress fracture and I thought life couldn't get much worse. Back then nothing could have been more depressing than being sidelined from training for several weeks. But a stress fracture seems so insignificant right now. I would prefer to have ten stress fractures than this horrible illness. Right now I don't care if I never run again. I just want to feel normal!

31 January 2007

Another day feeling like I am never going to get better. Life is just too hard right now. The fogginess seems to be getting worse and my legs are getting weaker. I struggled to walk from Bourke Street to Southbank to meet a friend — that's less than one kilometre. How can that be?

I had dinner at Mum and Dad's this evening, but I wish I had just stayed home. I was a miserable mess. I confessed to my parents that I don't know if I can go on any longer. It's all too hard. My mum walked out of the room crying. My parents are suffering just as much as me. How could I do this to them after everything they have done for me? They don't deserve it. I'm an awful, stubborn daughter who refused to listen.

My life sucks right now. I can't run, I don't want to eat because I will get fat. I am fat. Everything is making me fat and I can't burn it off. I'm hungry during the day and I know I should eat, but I just can't. And even if I did eat, who's to say I will get better?

I have nothing to look forward to. I know I pushed my body to the extreme, but does that really justify the adversity that my life has become?

7 February 2007

Over it, over it, over it! I am so sick of having to listen to patients complain about pain when I feel like shit. I had a patient come to see me this morning and she was going on and on about the pain in her knee. I felt like saying to her, 'Get over it. It's knee pain! At least you don't feel dizzy and drunk and unbalanced and have weird sensations in your legs twenty-four hours a day!'

*I don't know how much longer I can go on treating
patients. It's not that I don't care about them, it's just that
they don't realise how much worse things could be than just
having measly knee pain. Aagh, when is this nightmare going
to end?*

14 February 2007

*Valentine's Day. No boyfriend. No flowers — not even
from Brent. I think he has finally tried to move on and I'm
devastated. Exhausted, dizzy, foggy, unbalanced. Still feel like
I am living in a cloud.*

*Don't want to see friends. Don't feel like going out. It's
an effort to maintain a conversation. And I'm no fun to
be around. Who wants to be around a sulky, depressed,
frustrated person who feels like her life is crumbling?*

*It's so hard to pretend I'm happy, to make out that
everything is okay. I know I am neglecting my friends but right
now I don't care. I just want to curl up into a ball and close
my eyes like a foetus and not wake up until I feel well. Being
in bed with my eyes closed is the only time I can forget about
the horrible symptoms and feel vaguely normal.*

*I had more of this tight, squeezing feeling in my right leg
today, as if I am wearing bike pants that are far too tight.
My right leg still feels like it weighs a tonne and both my legs
feel like jelly. It feels like someone is pushing me over when I
walk, as if there is an invisible external force trying to push me
off balance.*

*I'm worried that I've made Mum sick from all the stress.
She has also been feeling heaviness in her right leg and it's
obviously quite bad because she went to see a doctor today.*

Friends asked me to join them for lunch later this week but I said no. There'd be too much tempting food. I feel so fat. The scales tell me I have only put on one kilogram since I stopped running but they must be lying. My bum is bigger than it has been in years and I have thunder thighs. I don't look like a marathon runner anymore.

I am counting every kilojoule. I haven't had pasta, bread, rice or potatoes for months. No processed foods, no sugar, no alcohol. How come other people can enjoy those foods and not get fat?

28 February 2007

It's been so long since I've seen Anna so when she told me she was coming down from Wangaratta and asked me to have lunch with her, I said yes. She is my best friend after all.

We had lunch in Lygon Street but it wasn't enjoyable. Not because of the company — I love spending time with Anna — but because I felt so crap the entire time. The brain fog was so extreme I could barely look at her. The strain on my eyes was too much. And I struggled to follow the conversation. I had to excuse myself twice to go to the bathroom, to give my eyes and my mind a break and to express my despair alone.

She realised something was really wrong when I returned red-eyed, my face puffy. She asked if there was anything she could do to help. I wish. I wish someone could do something to help me. But no-one can. It is so unfair that just a short catch-up with a friend is such an effort. Can life get any worse?

5 March 2007

I had a slightly better day today. My legs felt stronger and the tightness was not so severe. It is SUCH a relief when some of the symptoms ease. It gives me a slight glimmer of hope and for a second I can almost remember what it is like to feel normal again. I am so jealous of everyone who feels normal.

I want to tap people on the shoulder when I walk past them on the street and remind them of how lucky they are to have their health and to never take it for granted. I find myself looking at other people's legs, trying to remember how it feels to be normal, to feel connected to the rest of your body and in control of each step. Not to feel as though they weigh a tonne. And to not feel drunk all the time must be amazing.

The control I had over my body when I was running is but a distant memory. My body has deserted me. I don't know who or what is controlling my legs at the moment but it sure isn't me. I know it's my fault but I don't know how to reverse it. I know I should nourish my body more. I'm trying to eat more, I really am, but I feel like a pig. And I can't see how eating more would make a difference anyway.

Oh, I would do anything just to get out there and work up a sweat! My body just won't let me!

I saw Brent today for the first time in a few weeks. I don't know what's holding me back because I just love the time we spend together and I know he is still keen for us to get back together. I feel like I can be myself around him, I can't explain it but it just feels right, like we are meant to be.

2 April 2007
Dear Body,
I am sorry for the torture I have put you through. I sincerely
regret the gruelling training sessions, the endless hours on
the cross-trainer, sweating out kilograms of body fluids and
pushing every muscle to the absolute limit. I am sorry for not
fuelling you properly and for ignoring your pleas for more food.
I promise I will listen to you from now on. If you tell me you
don't feel like running, I won't force you to. If you tell me you
feel like sitting on the couch all day, that is where I will stay.
*   Please, Body, just give me one more chance. That is all I am*
asking for. I am trying so hard to nourish you with all sorts
of food but you have to understand the battle that is going
on in my head. It's a struggle. But I promise, if you give me
one more chance, I will look after you from now on. I will not
inflict any torture or pain on you. I would dearly love to run
again but if you do not wish to, I will respect this and I will
not push you to do so. I just want to feel healthy again.
*   Thank you for listening.*

'There can't be anything wrong with me!' I cried as I ran into Brent's arms.

It was April, the weekend before Easter. I had just run three kilometres. I hadn't broken any records, but it was further than I had run in over seven months. I had felt comfortable for most of it. I wouldn't say I felt strong, but there wasn't the weakness in my legs that had plagued me the past few months. I felt a little foggy in the head, but towards the end of the run, my head felt clearer than it had in a long time.

Small achievements such as these, which seemed impossible only two months earlier, assured me that there couldn't be anything seriously wrong and that I was on the way up. Although the run drained all my energy, I felt no worse than usual that evening. Trevor's treatment seemed to be working and maybe my body was considering giving me a second chance.

The afternoon of my three-kilometre achievement, there was another reason to celebrate. Brent and I became a couple again. It is often the case that something positive comes out of an unfortunate, challenging situation and one positive aspect of the past few months was that it had brought Brent and I closer together.

I found myself wanting to spend more and more time with him until I couldn't imagine life without him. That particular afternoon we were sitting on the beach while eating an ice cream, my one treat for the week, watching people play beach volleyball when out of nowhere I told him I wanted us to get back together. He almost dropped his ice cream as he leaned back and looked at me, unable to mutter a word for several seconds, a look of disbelief on his face. It wasn't the reaction I had expected.

'Are you sure this is what you want?' he asked after what seemed like minutes, still looking stunned.

'What do you mean?' I replied. 'I wouldn't be telling you this if I wasn't sure.'

'You have been resisting for so long. I find it hard to believe this is really how you feel.'

I finished off the last of my waffle cone, took his hands in mine and stared into his eyes. I took a deep breath. 'I have been thinking about it for a long time,' I began. 'This illness has made me realise there are so many more important things in life than running.

Things I have taken for granted the past few years: my health, my family, my friends ... and you. I have known all along that I want us to be together. I just wasn't sure if I was ready to make that commitment and I wanted to be one hundred per cent sure that I was before telling you. I can't imagine my life without you in it. Hun, I love you.'

Seconds of silence followed as he processed what I had said. Finally, a smile spread across his face. I could tell he didn't want to get too excited just yet. Instead, he was cautiously jubilant in case I changed my mind. But I wasn't going to change my mind. Not now, not ever. I leaned forward to kiss him and as our lips touched, I felt the same exhilarating feeling I had felt during our first kiss in Thailand five years earlier.

Over the next few weeks I gradually increased the distance and frequency I was running. I ran no more than five kilometres at a time and only on the days I didn't work so as to give myself time to recover. Thanks to Trevor's treatment my energy levels were definitely improving, however, all the other disturbing symptoms still remained. I vowed to look after my body but was still caught up in a battle with the incoherent voice in my head that forced me to continue counting every kilojoule that entered my mouth.

A five-kilometre run equates to approximately the number of kilojoules in a salad sandwich and I just couldn't bring myself to eat any more than that afterwards. I continued to avoid social gatherings where copious delicacies would threaten my willpower and put me at risk of exceeding my limited kilojoule allowance. On the rare occasions when I found myself surrounded by friends and food, I used the excuse that I had just eaten, wasn't hungry or was feeling a little nauseous. I was a nutritionist, and knew all too well that my actions were not providing my body with an optimum healing environment. With Brent now back in my life I was happier than I had been in a long time but the voice refused to relinquish control and this unwavering domination, which to some was viewed as sheer discipline, was a reflection of a severely troubled, self-absorbed young woman.

My energy levels continued to improve. By June 2007, a little over six months since I first went to see Trevor, I was working twenty-five hours a week and running eight kilometres, four times a week. My perpetual symptoms meant that running was far from enjoyable, but at least I was burning kilojoules.

By mid-July, almost exactly one year since the onset of my symptoms, my energy levels had returned to normal and it wasn't long before I was running every day. Regardless of how I felt, I was convinced that exercise made me feel better (at least psychologically) and forced myself out the door every morning. I chose to ignore the fact that I was falling back into the same trap that had made me so ill in the first place. My symptoms persisted too, making each day still a battle to get through.

I continued to see Trevor every couple of weeks. Even though he seemed at a loss to explain my continuing symptoms, as my energy levels had improved remarkably since I had started seeing him and I always felt more positive when I left his clinic. Despite this, the longer my symptoms remained, the more difficult it was to believe that one day I would feel normal. While previous MRIs on my brain and spinal cord had not revealed any abnormalities, I knew things may have changed. I was fed up with doctors and scared of what they might diagnose, but I needed to put my mind at ease, so I returned to my neurologist.

Dr Faraday did not appear surprised to see me at all. I felt like he knew something about my illness that he hadn't disclosed during my first visit. Maybe he had seen cases like mine on numerous occasions, patients who suffered for years before finally being given a diagnosis. Call it paranoia, but I couldn't help thinking the worst. He asked me how I was feeling. I was proud to tell him Trevor's treatment had improved my energy levels and that I was running regularly. He looked pleasantly surprised and told me he hadn't expected to hear that. Great, I thought. He expected me to tell him I was still struggling to get out of bed and could barely walk. Nothing like a bit of encouragement.

'But I am still experiencing horrible symptoms, which is why I have come back to see you. I am still constantly foggy, dizzy, unbalanced and I have disturbing, constricted feelings in my legs. I also have intense nerve-like pain shooting down my left leg. My right leg feels like it weighs a tonne and the last few days I have had severe pain in both feet first thing in the morning. I'm scared that one day I will wake up and not be able to walk,' I admitted.

After more questions and a brief physical assessment, he referred me for another MRI on my brain and spinal cord. The week between having the MRI and my follow-up appointment, my symptoms worsened, accentuating my stress and anxiety. I hadn't told my parents about returning to the neurologist, but because I hadn't changed my original contact details, they found out when they received a call from the clinic to confirm my follow-up appointment. Mum rang me immediately.

'I thought you were getting better?' she asked nervously. 'You're back running and your strength has improved.'

I was furious that the clinic had called my parents. They didn't need any more sleepless nights.

'I just want to be sure,' I replied. 'I am feeling a lot stronger and I have more energy, but I still have some nasty symptoms and I'm sick of them.'

I tried to sound positive but the tone in my voice revealed my nerves and anxiety. I was sick of lying and pretending everything was alright to my family, my friends, to everyone.

'I'll be okay. Please don't worry, Mum,' I said. 'I'll ring you after my appointment tomorrow. It will be at about two o'clock.'

I told her I loved her and hung up the phone. Not long after my brother rang me to wish me luck for my results. I had never heard him sound as concerned as during that phone call. He later told me that Mum had called him in tears after discovering I had returned to the neurologist. My illness was consuming my whole family and the angst they were enduring was all my fault. It was hard to swallow.

I sat behind a large desk in Dr Faraday's consulting room and watched as he opened my file, pulling out the report of my MRI. My hands were shaking and my heart raced. The temperature of the room suddenly increased. Seconds felt like minutes, minutes like hours. No matter how many times I was in this situation, the anticipation of receiving results didn't get any easier. The report could decide my future. Would I still be walking in a few years? Would I ever be able to have children? (This is not something I wanted at the time but I knew down the track that I would.) Would I ever feel like a normal person and be able to enjoy life again?

'The good news is that your results have come back normal,' he said. 'No abnormalities are evident.'

'Are you serious?' I managed to utter, as the bubble of angst and worry that had been building inside me for the past few weeks burst. I have never, ever bawled in front of a stranger as I did then. I couldn't contain myself.

'Sorry,' I sobbed, my head buried in my hands. 'I have been so worried.'

'It's okay,' he reassured me. 'It's normal to feel this way. You are going through a difficult time. Take a few deep breaths.'

I regained my composure.

'I don't think at this stage that there is any point doing more tests. The MRI you had last week is more sensitive than the ones you had previously. It picks up lesions in ninety-five per cent of cases. It's a great sign that your energy levels have returned and I think it's just a matter of time before you feel completely well again.'

This was far more reassuring than my last visit. I couldn't wipe the smile from my face as I left the clinic, overwhelmed but ecstatic with my results. I had pretty much exhausted all the necessary investigations. I wanted to scream to the world that it was just a matter of time until my body would heal and I would feel well again.

I rang my parents as soon as I walked out of the clinic. My mum answered the phone and the moment I heard her voice the waterworks were on again.

'I'm okay!' I managed to blurt out in between the tears. 'There's no need to worry, nothing is wrong.'

I could barely string a sentence together so I hung up and sent her a text message: 'All good. I'll call back later.'

2 September 2007

As I walked down the street today I gazed at people passing me and wondered what was going on in their lives. I wondered if they endured invisible suffering too. Were they living with silent symptoms like me?

It's amazing to think that every day we might walk past someone who has cancer, someone who has diabetes or someone who has heart disease. Others might have debilitating migraines, neck or back pain. Maybe they have just lost a loved one or they are in the middle of a divorce. Or maybe they are dizzy and foggy and feeling unbalanced. I'm sure there are many people out there who are — I just never thought I would be one of them

9 October 2007

Today is the two-year anniversary of my run at the Melbourne Marathon. I remember the exhilaration as I crossed the line and ran into the arms of family and friends — the best moment of my life.

I know I have to move on and accept I'm not a marathon runner any more and that my body does not want to run another marathon, but it's just so hard. I was so fit back then. I was lean. I had no body fat. I didn't feel guilty about having my treats on Sundays. These days I can't enjoy any food without feeling guilty.

That voice in my head just won't go away. I wish it would leave me alone. Right now I feel like I am at the lowest point in my life and am bringing my family down with me. Life is not worth living

15

Desperate

With serious neurological conditions having been ruled out, and feeling totally fed up with medical tests failing to provide answers, in between monthly visits to see Trevor, I embarked on a journey of natural therapies.

Over a period of five months I sought treatment and advice from over ten different healthcare practitioners, including a natural body healer, an acupuncturist, another naturopath, a Chinese medicine herbalist, a chiropractic neurologist and an Emotional Freedom Techniques (EFT) teacher. In addition, I also had an appointment with an immunologist and on his recommendation, a psychiatrist. After each initial assessment, I would brace myself for their verdict.

'Your qi is blocked. I will be able to help you unblock it with acupuncture.'

'Are you depressed? Depression can manifest as a range of symptoms including fatigue, brain fog and dizziness.'

'Your energy pathways are unbalanced. Weekly treatment will rebalance them and should eliminate your symptoms.'

'You need to believe you will get better. I can help you focus your mind on positive thoughts and healing. It will take several sessions, but it will happen.'

'Your hormone levels are unbalanced, which is the likely cause of your dizziness and fogginess. If we can balance the levels out again, you will feel great.'

No-one could tell me exactly how many sessions were required to resolve my symptoms. I was told on many occasions that since my condition was complex, they would need to see me several times before I would notice a difference. I persevered with most for five or six sessions but with no noticeable improvement, I moved on. It cost me a fortune but I was desperate. I was naive. I was gullible, easily convinced that each new therapy would work. Meanwhile, I continued to sink into my exercise obsession and kilojoule deprivation, unable to rise to the surface and see clearly. If only my vision hadn't been so limited by my addiction to exercise and a desire to stay lean, I would have saved thousands of dollars and endless hours searching for answers.

The immunologist left me feeling outraged. His tests failed to explain my symptoms so he concluded that I must be depressed and imagining the symptoms – he told me to see a psychiatrist. I couldn't believe what I was hearing. If I wake up feeling normal tomorrow, I will be the happiest person in the world! I wanted to yell at him. Depression is not the cause of my symptoms. Despite being sure his prediction couldn't have been further from the truth, I took his advice and saw a psychiatrist. I didn't want to regret not having tried every possible avenue.

The psychiatrist spent a total of thirty minutes questioning me before informing me we had run out of time and he would continue his assessment next time. He said I would need another two sessions before he was able to say if he could help me. I received an invoice in the mail a couple of days later for that initial session – three hundred dollars! I couldn't believe it. If I wasn't depressed before, I thought, I am now. I didn't return to see him.

The last straw in this alternative medicine journey from hell was my experience with a chiropractic neurologist who specialised in neurological pathways in the body. I still believed that there was a neurological element to my symptoms so I was confident it would be money well spent. For over an hour, Dr Taylor, a man of no more than forty with a rather abrupt manner which did little to ease my anxiety, drilled me with questions. By now my list of symptoms was nearly a page long:

- brain fog
- dizziness
- feeling drunk and unbalanced
- feeling as though I am being pushed over as I walk
- feeling like I am on a boat
- unable to concentrate
- right leg feels heavier than the left
- shooting pain down the back of left thigh
- occasionally feels as if something is in the bottom of my shoe
- tightness and heaviness in my legs
- feeling like someone is squeezing my thighs
- pins and needles in hands
- extreme coldness in hands and feet, sometimes they feel like ice to touch.

He conducted his initial assessment, which was similar to Trevor's. He assessed my voluntary motor function and coordination, which is controlled by the cerebellum, a small structure at the base of the brain. He then proceeded to hook me up to a specialised machine with approximately thirty electrodes connected to my head to assess the wave patterns in my brain and try to identify any dysfunction that could explain my symptoms. The entire assessment took two hours.

'It seems as though there is some neurological disturbance,' he started, a concerned frown on his face.

I could have told you that, I thought.

'A disruption in the wave patterns in your brain is likely to be contributing to your brain fog and feeling of being unbalanced,' he continued.

I wondered how this could be responsible for the strange sensations in my legs, but I refrained from asking. Just keep quiet and listen, I told myself. Stop trying to analyse everything.

'We need to retrain the brain and normalise the wave patterns. There is a specialised machine that I have used on many patients to help do this. It will take time and it will take some work on your behalf, but I think it is the answer you have been looking for.'

I've heard that before, I thought. I so desperately wanted to believe him but all I could think of was the endless times I had heard those words, only to be disheartened months and hundreds of dollars later. But I was keen to try it – after all, this may be the answer I was searching for – so he explained to me how to use the machine. I was horrified to discover the consultation cost two hundred and fifty dollars and the machine cost one thousand dollars per month to hire. I felt ill at the thought of having to fork out this amount after already having spent over five thousand dollars in medical bills in less than eighteen months, made more disheartening by the fact I was only working part time. But when I went to pay, the receptionist told me the bill had already been covered.

'I beg your pardon?' I replied.

'A lovely man with grey hair came in to pay it yesterday,' she said. 'His name was Rodney.'

I burst into tears, once again unable to hide my emotion. My dad had come to the clinic the day before to pay for the appointment and for the machine hire for four months in case that's what was recommended. The receptionist came around the front of the desk to comfort me. I was so ashamed.

My parents were desperate to see me happy again. I had been such a burden on them since the onset of my illness, emotionally and financially and yet, as always, they were going out of their way to help me. It upset me that I was so dependent on them. They didn't deserve any of this. I picked up the machine, thanked the lady, walked out and sobbed all the way home.

25 November 2007

I had a dinner party last night to celebrate my 28th birthday. It was the most fun I have had in a long time (which doesn't say much). Brent told me how wonderful it was to see me happy and having fun with my friends. That doesn't happen often these days. How can I enjoy other people's company when I don't enjoy my own? I made cookies, chocolate cake and cheesecake for dessert and I indulged in them all.

Thankfully the voice gave me a break last night so I felt no guilt devouring them but it was back again this morning so I went for a ten-kilometre run and then walked six kilometres. I know I haven't burnt off all those desserts and right now I feel a strong urge to walk another six kilometres.

Brent and I are planning a trip overseas next year. At least it's something to look forward to. I refuse to surrender to my symptoms and will continue this battle for as long as it takes. In the meantime I will NOT let it get in my way of doing anything.

I think we'll go to South America and maybe parts of the Middle East. I'd loved to meet my extended family in Israel.

Maybe a trip to Bethlehem will cure me. I can't wait to escape the monotony of life. And to spend money on something other than therapists.

21 December 2007

I came home from work today bawling, overwhelmed by the immense struggle it is just to get through each day. My outbursts are less frequent these days, probably two or three times per week now. Not because my symptoms are resolving, but because I am getting used to them.

I have been using the machine Dr Taylor recommended every night for over two months now. I have to connect it to my head and play computer games — using my mind instead of my hands to control the characters on the screen. It's frustrating because I don't really know what I'm doing and I don't feel like I'm controlling anything. There's been no improvement so far. Another big fat waste of money.

I'm still running most days but it's not enjoyable because I feel so shit. I know I have inflicted everything on myself and that I have only myself to blame, but I still don't know what to do to get better. I know I'm a little too lean still and I probably need to eat more but I don't want to get fat and in any case, I can't see how putting on weight is going to make these symptoms go away.

I was so distraught last night that I called my parents and they drove fifty minutes to give me a hug. I don't know what I would do without them. Brent has been amazing. He is my rock and I know he always will be. Not once has he or my parents said to me that this is my own fault or that I deserve what I am going through. They told me so many times that I was pushing my body too hard and I was too lean, but I was too stubborn to listen. There is nothing I can do and there will never be anything I can do to repay them for their endless love and support. All I can say to them is, 'Thank you. I love you very much.'

After three months of using the machine and three thousand dollars, my symptoms hadn't improved so I began doubting whether it was the solution I had been looking for. When I rang Dr Taylor to ask him whether he thought I should persevere, his reply infuriated me.

'It's up to you,' he said, matter-of-factly. 'It could take a few more months but no-one knows for sure. If you are willing to give it more time, you have a greater chance of getting better.'

I looked at the phone in utter disbelief. He might as well have told me I was just another number who had walked through the door of his clinic and he didn't really care what I did. When I told him I wanted to stop treatment and I asked for a refund for the machine hire for the fourth month, he harshly informed me a refund was against the clinic's policy and he had to get off the phone because he had a patient waiting. I let him hear every single bit of what I was thinking. I hung up in absolute despair, feeling more distraught than ever. Things couldn't get much worse.

When I reflect on those few months, on the person I was then, I am understanding of myself, but am still surprised by my lack of introspection. I spent countless hours and thousands of dollars begging others to unravel the cause of my symptoms and miraculously solve my problems. Yet it was all so simple and clear. I had the power to change my life but I was unwilling to admit my mistakes, and ultimately, to face them.

16

2008 Adventure

1 January 2008

Disastrous start to the new year. We went to St Kilda pier with Brent's friends but I felt dizzy and unbalanced all night and my legs were so tight and constricted. I know I wasn't much fun to be around but all I wanted was a bit of compassion and sympathy.

Brent wouldn't have a bar of it. He just kept telling me to be positive. Easy for him to say. He doesn't understand how I feel. No-one does. We ended up having a huge fight. I know he doesn't deserve a girlfriend who complains all the time. I know I bring him down when I am like that but sometimes I just need to take my frustration out on someone.

He sent me a text message today saying he doesn't know how long he can keep going on like this. There is absolutely no point feeling sorry for myself but I just feel so trapped, as if there is no way out of this mess. I am drowning, screaming inside to be fished out from this bottomless ocean and although there are people around me trying to help, no-one can pull me out of these treacherous waters because no-one can fully understand how deep and how torturous these waters are. How can they? I sound crazy when I describe what I'm feeling.

I forced myself to run ten kilometres this morning in 35° heat. I felt horrible but at least I know I have burnt some *energy today. And I only had a piece of toast for breakfast so no guilt there. I'm feeling a bit more positive now. I have to believe that this year will be a good one. I will be completely cured, rid of all my symptoms! Bring on the new year and a new me!*

I was on a rollercoaster of emotions. I was desperate one minute, feeling alone and misunderstood, the next upbeat and positive, excited at the prospect of feeling well. Every morning when I woke up I lay with my eyes closed for several minutes, imagining and trying so hard to believe that I would feel completely normal when I opened them.

Now that my energy was back, the voice in my head forced me to exercise every day. I wanted to rebel and tell the voice that I didn't care, that I was no longer a marathon runner and probably never would be so there was no need to look like one. But I felt powerless against the tremendous compulsion to burn as many kilojoules as possible.

Feeling unwell or tired was not an excuse. Just push through, the voice nagged when I thought about having a day off. Don't be weak. I continued counting every kilojoule I consumed to ensure I didn't exceed my limited allowance. I was eating so little during the day that I often woke during the night with hunger pains. Some nights they were so intense that I couldn't get back to sleep if I didn't eat so I crawled into the kitchen in a semi-conscious state and rummaged through the cupboards to find something to satisfy my hunger. A muesli bar, a tub of yogurt or a bowl of cereal usually sufficed.

These midnight snacks became a habit. I was like a baby waking during the night for a feed. As I had done a couple of years prior, I began to eat less during the day to save kilojoules for the night feeds. If I exceeded my intake one day, I worked for twice as long the next.

By February 2008, despite persisting symptoms, I was running ten to twelve kilometres, seven times per week and going to the gym at least three times per week. Any less than ten kilometres and I felt like I was wasting my time. To my delusional mind sixty kilometres per week was not much at all. I also cycled to work but I didn't consider that exercise. I was beginning to overdo it again, exercising at all costs. Many people warned me again but I didn't listen – there was nothing I could do to stop.

Every night I read the quotes on my wall, focusing on the third one. 'Remove physiological stress from the body and the body does what it is designed to do. It heals itself.' I knew what it was telling me, but I continued to believe I was different. Brent could clearly see that I had embarked on the same journey of self-destruction, despite my efforts to hide it.

'Have you not learnt your lesson?' he said to me one night when I told him I was off for a run for the second time that day. 'What more does your body need to do for you to listen to it?'

'It's a nice, balmy night and I feel like running,' I replied. 'Is there anything wrong with that?' What I really meant was, 'I ate a piece of cake at work today. I need to burn it off.'

'Yes there is,' he said firmly. 'Do you want to end up like you were a couple of years ago, not being able to get out of bed? How can you expect your symptoms to disappear if you don't look after your body?'

'I feel crap anyway, so what difference will an extra run make?'

I replied. I wanted to reason with him, to display a normal mental state and the capacity for logical thought, but the voice was pushing me out the door.

12 February 2008

It's over eighteen months since the onset of these horrible symptoms. I have been plagued with constant ill health for OVER A YEAR AND A HALF. I can't believe this has gone on for so long.

I would never have imagined that I would take an entire year off training. I know I'm lucky to be running at all, but how can I be content running only eight to ten kilometres a few times a week when I feel so bad? And I am so slow it's embarrassing.

I'm so over feeling like this all the time. I'm so over pretending everything is okay when it's not. I'm sick of people not understanding how I feel. It's all too hard. I know I should be grateful that nothing serious has been diagnosed. I am. Really, I am thankful. But I just want to feel normal again.

I know a lot of people think it's all in my head. I wish everyone could experience what I am feeling, just for one day. Just so they could understand what I am going through. Then I wouldn't feel so alone.

19 February 2008

I have spent so much money on natural therapies but nothing is helping. I'm still seeing Trevor every few weeks but if someone could guarantee they would eliminate my symptoms I would hand over $10 000. Or more. I am desperate and I just don't know what to do anymore.

I don't know how much longer I can go on. I feel fat and lazy. I'm only running about sixty kilometres each week. That's less than half what I used to run. Thank goodness for this overseas trip that Brent and I are planning. I actually can't believe he wants to travel with me. I'm far from fun to be around at the moment. But thank goodness he is happy to, I really need something else to think about, something to look forward to. And I plan to leave all these horrible symptoms behind.

25 May 2008

Finally the time has come to live my life again. To explore exciting new countries, experience different cultures and meet interesting people. It's time to leave my symptoms behind, to stop spending money on medical appointments and forget about the past two years of my life. No medical appointments for at least five months. I am so excited to be travelling again, but I am a bit apprehensive that my symptoms will ruin my trip. I keep telling myself that my symptoms didn't board the plane — they stayed home.

I am going to be one hundred per cent and it'll be as great as any of our previous adventures. Thailand, France, Israel, Jordan, Columbia, Peru, Bolivia, Chile, Argentina, Brazil and USA here we come!

Our first stop was Bangkok. I had been there many times so I knew where to find suitable accommodation: something clean and cheap. The day after we arrived, we went to the Bangkok prison in a town called Nonthaburi. We were visiting Abdullah, a prisoner from Ghana who I had met during my first trip to Thailand in

2000. He was in prison for drug trafficking and was on death row, but proclaimed his innocence. A group of backpackers had given me his name as one of many foreign prisoners who go months or years without visitors, abandoned by their families who live thousands of kilometres away.

My first visit was an amazing, memorable experience and we'd kept in touch with regular letters. He'd told me that receiving my letters was the highlight of his week and a welcome break to the monotony of prison life. He had no access to computers or telephones, so handwritten letters were the only option. He shared a small room with twenty inmates, many of them murderers, and was fed two small bowls of watery rice each day. Innocent or not, Abdullah's life in prison was a living hell.

It was my fourth visit to the prison but I was still covered in goose bumps as I entered the gates. Walking down the first aisle was creepy as murderers dressed in blue hospital-like gowns, their ankles tied by chains, glanced at us. They were waiting for loved ones to pay them a visit. It felt surreal. Glass separated the prisoners and visitors so the only way to communicate was by telephone.

Brent and I had a good chat with Abdullah – about movies, sport, world news, life inside the prison, his sentence and his hope to be sent back to Ghana – before the bell rang and we were ordered to leave. We left him with some food, including nuts, bars, chocolate and fruit.

Since that visit I have not heard from him. I wrote him a letter at the end of 2008 but it was the first time I did not receive a reply. Whether he was granted his wish and sent back to Ghana or whether he succumbed to the harsh Thai laws, I do not know.

4 June 2008

Oh Paris, jolie Paris, a modern city hidden behind beautiful old fronts. With its old buildings bordering the river and the chic Champs Elysées. You can hear the shrill calls of swallows gliding swiftly through the sky as you cross a bridge over the River Seine, which provides a perfect backdrop to the ancient Notre Dame Cathedral. It's been over three years since I was here and it is great to see my family again. We went to the French Open today. Through his work at the Australian Open, overseeing player services, Brent was given passes into the players' lounge and access to all courts. The sun was out, the sky was blue, the world's best graced the courts.

I felt okay for the first half of the day before the dizziness and unsteadiness kicked in. My legs are feeling quite constricted and jelly-like, but I'm trying to ignore it. I won't let these symptoms ruin our trip.

I ate three crepes today. I feel disgusting, but at least I went for a twelve kilometre run this morning and I'll run again tomorrow. It's not every day I have the opportunity to enjoy delicious French food!

18 June 2008

We arrived in Jerusalem today, exhausted after very little sleep on the plane from Paris. We arrived at 9 am and mustered up the energy to walk around this ancient city. We followed the four-kilometre wall surrounding the old city of Jerusalem, walked down narrow alleyways and explored colourful markets. There is a magical quality about this city that I have never seen before. Its towering stone walls and ancient buildings combined with the city's dynamic history woven with war and peace, love and hate, destruction and resurrection makes this city so unique.

I'm not feeling too bad, slightly dizzy and unbalanced and my legs definitely don't feel normal. Dinner was torture tonight. I did no exercise today but had to accept everything that was put on my plate because I didn't want to be rude and offend anyone. It was delicious — an array of meats, pasta, salads and other creamy delicacies that I had never tasted before — but I couldn't enjoy it. I still feel guilty.

Off to bed now. Lots of energy to burn tomorrow.

25 June 2008

Today has been one of those days. I'm well and truly over it. I just want to feel NORMAL! We swam in the Dead Sea today — or rather floated due to its extremely high salt content. It is situated at the lowest point of dry land on earth, more than four hundred metres below sea level so it was hot and I think this accentuated my symptoms. I was feeling so unbalanced and when I got out of the water, it felt as if someone was tying a tourniquet around my thighs.

Brent and I had a fight today all because of my stupid symptoms. I don't know why he continues to stick by me. He told me I am ruining his trip by complaining all the time and he can't take it anymore. I was inconsolable. I don't want to ruin everything for him but at the same time keeping everything locked up inside me with no-one to talk to is so hard.

30 June 2008

South America. We are finally here. After hearing endless stories from Mum, Dad and my brother, who have all spent months travelling around this fascinating continent, it is our turn to experience the magic and wonder of what it has to offer.

We landed in Bogota, Columbia, two days ago. I can understand why we were warned of pickpockets and told to remove anything valuable. There are plenty of seedy-looking people around and I definitely wouldn't want to walk alone at night. We have this strange, eerie feeling of being watched and are constantly looking over our shoulders. Despite this feeling of unease, the locals we have met are very friendly.

All is good between Brent and I after we had a chat and I told him I'll do everything to be more positive from now on so we can both enjoy this adventure.

4 July 2008

Wow, what a day! We arrived in Lima, Peru just before midnight and thought better of venturing into an unknown city with no accommodation booked, so we spent the night at the airport. We found a quiet corner in the arrivals lounge and slept on the floor.

At 7 am we took a bus into the city, but it hadn't occurred to us that we would be in the middle of peak-hour traffic. Crammed into a small bus like sardines in a tin, our backpacks on, not knowing where we were going, was as much of a challenge as getting useful directions from the locals, who speak no English. The traffic was horrendous, cars weaving in and out of lanes around the hundreds of buses, the constant sound of horns blaring.

Between Brent and I, our Spanish is non-existent, but I had convinced myself that my near-fluent French would be enough to get me by. I have been advised to say the word

in French and add an 'o' on the end. So far that advice is
proving useless: people just stare at me with a blank gaze.
Thankfully we have a Spanish phrase book. I'm not exactly
stringing sentences together but it's enough to get by.

After discovering we were heading in the wrong direction
we changed buses and finally arrived in the city square. We
wandered the narrow, cobbled streets for nearly an hour under
a dark threatening sky before finding a bed for the night in
a cheap hostel hidden down a small alley. After handing over
thirty Peruvian Nuevo Sols (approximately eleven Australian
dollars) we went straight to our room, dropped our bags on
the floor and collapsed on the bed. Although we could feel
every spring in the mattress and the pillows were as hard as
a rock (budget accommodation!), we both fell asleep.

After exploring the capital city of Lima for a couple of days, we took
an eight-hour bus trip to Huaraz, a beautiful town to the north.
The town was surrounded by snow-covered mountain peaks, their
monstrosity making them appear far closer to the town than they
were. The crystal blue sky and the rays of the sun glistening on the
mountains provided a perfect backdrop for the picturesque town
which was filled with narrow, paved lanes and pointy rooftops. The
mountains, intriguing and enticing, easily convinced us to book a
trek for the following day.

'Have you done any trekking through snow before?' the man
selling the trek asked.

'No, we haven't,' Brent replied.

'So I'm guessing you haven't worn crampons before?'

'What are they?' I asked.

'They are the shoes you need to wear to trek through snow. Some areas are icy and without them you would not have sufficient grip.'

Never before had I trekked through snow, let alone snow so icy that it required special footwear.

He continued, 'Have you spent time here in Huaraz acclimatising to the high altitude?'

We had gone from fifteen hundred metres to just over three thousand metres overnight, higher than we had ever been before.

'Not really,' Brent replied. 'We arrived this morning. We spent the last four days in Lima. We both feel fine though.'

The man looked at us with mysterious dark eyes, for what seemed to be an eternity. I couldn't quite work out what he was thinking or what he was trying to unravel with his gaze. I expected to hear we did not meet the requirements and wouldn't be allowed on the trek. No experience trekking through snow or wearing crampons and most importantly, we had been at three thousand metres for less than twenty-four hours. I was therefore surprised with his response.

'Okay, everything sounds good. We can get you on a trek tomorrow. You'll have a private guide. If you do the two-day trek you will leave here at eight o'clock in the morning, trek to four thousand seven hundred metres where you will set up camp. At one o'clock in the morning you will trek to the summit, which is at six thousand metres. Your guide will carry all the equipment and food. These are some of the views you will see.'

The photos he showed us were breathtaking. Exactly what you'd expect to see in *National Geographic*. I was surprised (and relieved) that he hadn't asked us about our medical history before deciding whether we were fit to attempt the climb. But this was Peru.

Salespeople are not renowned for taking necessary precautions and your health is not their concern. If I had turned up with one leg he probably would have let me begin the trek. He hadn't yet mentioned the price and I knew we had to be careful not to be ripped off.

'What is the price of the trek?' I asked.

'A two-day trek is one hundred and fifty dollars per person. A three-day trek is two hundred dollars per person. That includes all food, transport, accommodation, equipment and a private guide. You will need the crampons and sleeping bags suitable for temperatures of minus ten to minus fifteen degrees as it will plummet to well below zero at night. We provide you with only the best equipment, free of charge.'

One night out in freezing temperatures sounded challenging enough, but two nights? I didn't think I could prepare myself for that.

'Will we reach higher altitude if we go on the three-day trek?' I asked. I wanted to conquer the highest mountain I could.

'No,' the man replied. 'You will reach the same summit on both treks but the three-day trek allows you to climb more slowly so you reach high altitude more gradually. You'll probably suffer less altitude sickness if you do it over three days.'

It was a no-brainer. Lower cost, only one night out in the freezing cold and the same goal accomplished. I turned to Brent who had 'I-don't-know-if-we-should-do-this' sprawled across his face.

'The two-day trek sounds good?' I asked rhetorically, ignoring his look of concern and giving him little choice but to agree.

'I don't know if this is a good idea,' he said. 'Your health is not one hundred per cent and we haven't had any experience climbing. We haven't acclimatised either. Do you really think it's a smart thing to do?'

Regardless of whether I thought it was smart, the challenge had been laid out in front of me and the idea of conquering this mountain was firmly engrained in my conscience. Whether it was running a sub-three-hour marathon, completing an assignment, writing a book or climbing a mountain, if a goal is set before me, I make sure I accomplish it. Anything less is considered failure. I knew attempting the climb wouldn't be the safest thing to do but my energy levels and strength were fine. This and a strong mind were surely all that was needed to conquer the mountain.

'We'll be fine,' I said, 'I think it will be good for me. It will give me something else to think about other than my symptoms. My energy levels are fine at the moment. I think we can do it.'

'You don't want to wait a few days to acclimatise?' Brent asked.

'We don't really have time to stay here a few days,' I said, aware of the enormity of the continent and the slow pace of travel. We only had three months in South America and there was so much to see.

'What would we do here for several days anyway? It's a tiny town that can be seen in a day. I don't want to be waiting around for several days with nothing to do. We'll get bored,' I insisted.

'OK, if you insist,' Brent said. 'But I think it's crazy.'

The man at the desk was listening to our conversation and a gracious smile spread across his face. Two more customers. He could probably finish work early. One hundred and fifty dollars is a lot of money in Peru; roughly three weeks of budget accommodation or seventy meals. We handed over three hundred dollars, collected a hand-written receipt and spent the next hour trying on clothes and shoes to help us endure the treacherous, freezing conditions.

We left town at around nine o'clock in the morning – Brent and I, our guide and a German tourist named Herbert. We weren't impressed to have a companion after being promised (and paying for) a private guide, but there was no point arguing. We were driven to four thousand metres and began trekking. It was a glorious day. The sun's rays warmed our bodies and complemented the gorgeous scenery, adding to the serenity of the experience.

We trekked for three hours to four thousand seven hundred metres carrying our own fifteen-kilogram backpacks (after being told our guide would carry everything) nibbling on snacks as we went. When our guide announced that we had reached our destination camp, Brent and I looked at each other in shock, both a little nervous. There was no actual camping site – just a small space on the edge of a cliff. Our guide instructed us to find the flattest piece of land, in between rocks and shrub, and to start pitching our tent while he began cooking dinner for us. There was no point arguing and the sun would be setting in a few hours so we obediently set to work.

We ate dinner at five thirty. The menu comprised only pea soup, hardly enough to fuel our bodies for the trek ahead. At least I didn't have to worry about consuming too many kilojoules. By six o'clock the sun had set and the temperature was nearing zero so we climbed into our tent and crawled into our sleeping bags. It took over an hour to begin feeling my toes and another hour to feel my hands. For five hours Brent and I lay awake, trying to use each other's body warmth to generate heat, only getting colder as the temperature outside plummeted into the negatives. My lips stung, my teeth chattered and my back ached as I felt the cold, hard, uncomfortable ground underneath me. Brent was shivering uncontrollably.

By eleven o'clock I had finally begun to thaw out but had the urge to go to the toilet. There was no way I was getting out of my sleeping bag and exposing my bare skin to the freezing air outside. I forced myself to hold on. The two hours that followed were the longest of my life. We both tried to sleep but to no avail. Every now and then I felt breathless and was forced to sit up. Brent started shivering then sweating, with periods of hallucinations in between. He complained of a splitting headache and struggled to move his body. What on earth have we got ourselves into? I thought.

The fact that we were perched on the edge of a cliff and medical help was nearly two thousand metres below was difficult to erase from my mind. Our guide was no doctor and wasn't carrying any oxygen. I could hear Brent breathing heavily and when I switched on the torch I saw his eyes were watering. Our bodies were resisting the high altitude and freezing temperature but there was nothing we could do. We would both have to tough this night out. Was this supposed to be fun? I thought.

An hour past midnight it was time to venture out and attempt our trek to the summit. Brent was still suffering the harsh effects of high altitude and couldn't move. I told him I would stay with him.

'No, you go,' he said to me. 'At least one of us has to make it to the summit.'

'Are you sure?' I replied. 'I don't want to leave you here all alone. We're in the middle of nowhere and there's no-one around.'

'Yes, I'm sure. There's nothing you can do anyway. Go for it. I know you can do it.'

I unzipped the tent and stepped outside to a huge gust of wind, the ice-cold air finding its way through my layers of clothing and piercing every bone in my body.

We began the trek – myself, Herbert and our guide. Each step was burdensome but for the first few hours, other than occasional breathlessness and feeling lightheaded, I didn't feel too bad. The darkness proved a blessing. It was such a steep climb that being able to see ahead would have been intimidating and provided an even greater mental challenge. I concentrated on taking one step at a time as we wallowed up vast, tilted snowfields. Over some areas I had to plunge my ice pick into the frighteningly steep snow just to be able to take another step forward.

After over six hours of the most physically demanding challenge I have ever experienced, the sun began to rise. On the other side of the mountain, it did nothing to warm us, but did strengthen my determination to reach the summit. Our increased visibility made me acutely conscious of the lethal drop to the right. I knew if I stepped too far on the fragile crest, I could plunge to my death.

With one hundred metres to the top to go, Herbert collapsed, face down in the snow. He dragged himself up, looking as white as the snow surrounding us, and tried to take another step. We were in soft snow and sank to our knees with each step. Herbert collapsed again ten minutes later and then again five minutes after that.

My hands were still numb and my lips stung but I felt well enough to continue. I wanted to keep going and reach the summit as quickly as possible so I could head back to camp to see Brent. I thought about him lying in the tent, praying he had survived the night. What if he hadn't? He had stood by me for so long, in good and poor health, he had supported me in every way and this was how I repaid him? I suddenly felt like I had been punched in the stomach and I thought I was going to be sick. At that moment I wished I had never left that tent. In fact I wished we had never decided to go on this trek. But I knew that all I could do right now was pray that he was still alive.

However despite being desperate to get to the summit, there were rules to abide by (which hadn't been explained to us). As the three of us were attached by a thick rope to prevent us falling off the edge of the cliff in case we misplaced our step, I was prohibited from going ahead alone. Towards the end Herbert was only managing five steps in between each halt, before slowly gathering the energy to drag himself back up. Each time he face planted in the snow, I felt a strong pull of the rope attached to my waist and a couple of times it nearly pulled me down.

I was furious, especially because we had paid for a private guide so we could go at our own pace. The effects of thin air started to weigh me down with less than one hundred metres to go. My breathing became loud and laboured and each step was a tremendous effort as I sank knee-deep into the soft snow. I looked up ahead. The summit was within reach but the incline incredibly steep. My steps became increasingly slow, my breathing more laboured as I took in three deep breaths per step. Come on, I thought. You're almost there. You can do this. The last hundred metres should have taken about thirty minutes, but with Herbert almost collapsing with every step, it took just over an hour.

After more than seven hours trekking in freezing temperatures and drawing on every ounce of psychological and physical strength, we reached the summit. I looked around. It was early morning so we enjoyed luminous clarity – endless snow-covered mountains surrounded us for as far as we could see, the sky bluer than I had ever seen it before. It felt like we were on the apex of a white roof, the point at which you can't go any higher. I had just conquered the greatest challenge of my life. What a feeling.

The breathtaking views were tempered by the sense that the long descent awaited and the air was vanishingly thin so we stayed at the summit for less than five minutes – enough time to capture the moment on camera – before turning around and, facing the wind, forcing our bodies to carry on down. Heading back to camp, my body began to thaw out but I started to feel the effects of the tremendous climb. Every muscle ached. I could feel blisters all over my feet and my boots dug into my shins as I raced down the steep slopes. What took us seven hours to climb up took a little over two hours to run down. When we reached camp, I ran straight over to our tent to find Brent lying down, thankfully looking more comfortable than nine hours earlier.

'You're alive!' I exclaimed as I threw myself into his arms. 'How are you feeling?'

'A bit better,' he replied. 'How was it?'

'Unbelievable,' I replied quietly, my voice shaking from the tremendous relief at finding Brent alive. I left it at that. I could fill in the details later.

I hadn't eaten anything in over twelve hours but had burned more energy than during a marathon. Pea soup was all that had been packed so it had to suffice as our recovery meal. After hurriedly eating a bowl of it, we began the teo-hour trek back down to four thousand metres, where our driver was waiting to drive us back into the town. It had been thirty hours since we left Huaraz and I can confidently say that I have never faced such physical and mental challenges in such a short period of time. Having thanked our guide, we returned our equipment and went straight to our hotel room where we both collapsed on the bed. I fell asleep with a smile on my face, satisfied with my accomplishment. I had just completed the most physically and emotionally challenging experience of my life, all on very limited kilojoules.

Although I have fond memories of the trek, what we did was audacious but extremely foolish. We were ignorant to the effects of high altitude and were extremely fortunate not to suffer dire consequences. To go from Lima, at fifteen hundred metres to the summit at six thousand metres, in less than forty-eight hours, carries the risk of cerebral oedema and haemorrhage – which is potentially fatal. I can also hardly believe that my focus on reaching the summit was so absolute that I had left Brent alone in the tent. My overriding desire to test my body's physical limits and achieve my goals at all costs made me oblivious to how selfish I was. Not only was I obviously prepared to see the summit on my own rather than share the experience with my partner, but my focus on the challenge ahead distracted me from the potentially fatal path I embarked on and the serious risks to Brent's health – and life – involved in leaving him on his own. It is almost impossible to comprehend that I did this and I still carry a feeling of guilt years later.

15 July 2008

Here we are in La Paz, Bolivia. I've felt absolutely terrible since the trek – tired, dizzy, foggy, unbalanced – but what did I expect? Brent has recovered from the effects of high altitude but he felt like resting today. I rested this morning but by lunchtime I was feeling lazy so I went for a walk on my own and stumbled across San Pedro prison. It's not as if I have always had a strong interest in prisons and prisoners but after such an eye-opening experience visiting the prison in Thailand, I thought I would try to get in and I did! What an amazing experience.

I sat with five other foreigners in the room of one of the inmates. While explaining his ordeal of being caught with a kilogram of heroin strapped to his body last year he gave us vodka and whisky and described how he smuggles drugs into the prison from the outside through a small hole in the roof. He talked about his wife and two children in South Africa; they've only visited him once.

He said if he had his time again he wouldn't change a thing — he was making good money smuggling drugs into different countries and believed you only live once so you have to make the most of it. I'm not sure I agree with him after seeing the atrocity of his living conditions! He took us on a tour of the prison and we met a few children who live with their fathers, who are inmates. It was like a movie. Such a creepy, chilling afternoon.

Tomorrow we are taking a bike ride down the most dangerous road in the world. Just another challenge? Yes. Adventurous? Yes. Stupid? Some would say yes to that, too!

16 July 2008

We survived the bike ride down the most dangerous road in the world! My ears were popping the entire way down!

We took a bus to 4700 m altitude then rode twenty-one kilometres down to 3600 m, then another 38 km to 1200 m. The sheer drop to one side meant that one slip up and we were over the edge; the small, stoned memorials on the side of the road, some decorated with photos and flowers, were a

bleak reminder of the travellers from around the world who
had lost control of their bikes and lost their lives.

When we arrived at the bottom of the mountain we were
served an array of different foods for lunch but I stuck to the
salads and vegetables. As we were driven back to the city
by minibus, the sun was setting and a thick blanket of fog
made it impossible for the driver to see the twists and turns in
the road. For the entire three-and-a-half-hour trip I was terrified
and I know everyone else was too. I have never, ever, been so sure
I was going to die. We clapped when we got to the top of the
mountain, thankful and relieved that we were still alive.

I'm still feeling my horrible symptoms every second of every
day but at least we are living life to the fullest!

5 August 2008

Argentina. Beautiful Argentina, diverse with its pristine
beaches, lush, dense forests, abundant mountains, dry, barren
deserts and mixed cultures. This is what we have read about it
and we're hoping to see some of it ourselves.

I'm trying to cheer myself up after another huge fight with
Brent. He is fed up with my sombre moods. I've been blaming
everything on him lately too, which doesn't help. He ended
up storming out of our hotel room this afternoon leaving me
feeling paralysed — in such shock that for a few minutes I
felt like I couldn't move. We are in a very small town at the
moment — there isn't too far to go — so I know he'll be back
... I hope.

I just wish he would try to understand, just for one second,
what it's like to feel drunk twenty-four hours a day. To dread
walking to dinner, knowing that I'm going to feel unbalanced

and constricted in my legs. He just doesn't get it. He says
he does, but he has no idea. How could he? My symptoms
sound crazy.

Yes, I am feeling sorry for myself right now. I feel so alone.
I'm so over it.

11 August 2008

After visiting the ferocious, gushing Iguaçu falls, surrounded
by lush green landscape and thick jungle, we have just spent
three days camping in the Pantanal, the largest wetland
spanning Brazil, Bolivia and Paraguay and over two hundred
thousand square kilometres, dense with wildlife, sparse of
people and towns.

We fished for and cooked up piranhas for lunch, went
horse riding and found ourselves just a metre from a caiman
(in the same family as an alligator). We slept in hammocks
and woke up to the sound of hundreds of birds. It really was
the true Brazilian experience.

I ran each day for at least forty minutes, but because of
the heat I had to run before 6 am. Everyone else thought I
was crazy for getting up so early and yes part of me knew
I was too, but I haven't had many opportunities to run so
I have to take every chance I get. We have done a lot of
walking so I don't think I have put on any weight, but that
voice in my head has not left me alone this entire trip.

'Don't eat too many kilojoules' – 'No, I haven't.'

'Run every chance you get' – 'Yes, I have run whenever
possible.'

'You are eating a lot of ice cream and if you don't burn it
off you will get fat!' – 'I am doing everything I can to burn it

off so shut up!'

Aagghh! Go away, voice. Leave me alone and let me
live. I feel trapped, a prisoner in my own body and a guard
watching my every move; taking note of every single piece of
food I put into my mouth.

I wish it would leave me alone.

14 August 2008

Rio de Janeiro. What a fabulous city!

We arrived in this hot, dry city yesterday morning after a
twenty-two-hour bus trip. There is definitely a Latin American
feeling to the place and I don't think this city ever slows
down — people are everywhere and they never stop moving.
We ended up walking for over three hours, down main roads,
through small narrow streets, occasionally having to step over
sewerage canals, just to find a hotel. Why didn't we get a
cab into the city? Because we are stubborn. Or rather, I am
stubborn. Taking a cab is cheating. Why would I take a cab
when I can walk for three hours and burn kilojoules? Brent
reluctantly but bravely endured the hot sun beating down on
us as we carried over 20 kg on our backs and roamed the
streets. All because I refused to take a cab. We eventually
found a small, dingy hostel that will be our home for the
next couple of weeks. The room has a bed and a table in it.
The shower and toilet are outside. I was excited about the
communal kitchen and we finally had a home-cooked meal
last night.

We spent the day today wandering the streets, exploring
all that this cosmopolitan city has to offer. The beautiful
Ipanema and Copacabana beaches, the elegant boutiques

and colourful markets. We only got a small taste of the vibrant nightlife when we went out for dinner tonight. Tomorrow we plan to ride the cable car up to Sugarloaf (Pão de Açúcar) that over looks the beautiful bay.

27 August 2008

What a fantastic couple of weeks exploring this fascinating city. The drug-infested favelas are out of this world, many of them close to collapsing. Electrical wires protrude from each and kids openly do drug deals in broad daylight. Copacabana beach is full of life, with locals dressed in little more than white G-strings, pursuing various forms of exercise — beach volleyball, running, swimming, aerobics. Vendors wander up and down the white sand all day, selling anything from bikinis to towels to sunglasses, hats and beer, trying to make a living off the crowds of people basking in the sun. Hundreds of small restaurants, cafés and bars line the beachfront, their aromatic, tempting smells drifting for miles. The people are so diverse and extremely friendly.

Tomorrow I'll be heading north to Salvador on my own. Brent is off to New York to spend time with his brother and I'll meet him there next week.

I'm so used to travelling with him that I'm a little worried I'll be lonely. Come on, toughen up!

31 August 2008

Wow, Salvador is such an exciting, vibrant city, full of character with its small cobbled streets in amongst a backdrop of brightly coloured colonial buildings — reds, yellows, oranges — that have been standing for over a hundred years. It has

an energy and unadorned beauty that I have not seen in
any other city. The new part of Salvador is full of residential
neighbourhoods and shopping megaplexes which I am finding
quite alienating. The old part represents the descendants of
African slaves who have preserved their heritage through
music, religion, food and dance traditions.

The locals are extremely friendly and easygoing and
love sharing their exotic dancing and music skills. It's not
everywhere you walk down the street in the middle of the
afternoon to the sound of drums pounding out powerful
rhythms, the locals singing and dancing, displaying vibrant
costumes. Everyone has so much rhythm here, it is so cool.
The plaza was alive tonight with groups performing capoeira
(a traditional form of martial arts) while the scent of acarajé
(bean and shrimp fritters) filled the evening air.

I found myself at the Mardi Gras yesterday. That sure
was an eye opener. The physique of some of those men
was formidable — their tall, sculpted, bronzed bodies and
prominent six-packs impossible to ignore, their erotic moves
startling. I was pickpocketed at some stage during the
afternoon but it was my own stupid fault for carrying a
backpack on my back with money in the front pocket.

I have found the best ice-creamery just down the street
from my hostel. The ice cream is served in fresh, warm wafer
cones and is so creamy, it's tantalising. They have an array
of flavours from cookies and cream to mango to peppermint
to guava. And the serves are BIG. I'm really watching my
kilojoule intake during the day so I can have one at night
without feeling too guilty. And yes, voice, I've been running
10 km and walking at least 15 km every day!

13 September 2008

*I am exhausted after a hectic week in New York. We stayed
with Brent's brother in Brooklyn Heights and went to
Broadway, the basketball, the baseball, the opera. We visited
Central Park, Times Square, went for several runs over the
Brooklyn Bridge, shopped in Soho, walked past Wall Street
and dined at the 'W' hotel. Sounds like a fabulous week —
which in a way it was and it was great to spend time with
Brent's brother who I had not seen in over three years — but
I have felt so drained all week, the dizziness and fogginess
worse than I can remember, that every day all I wanted to
do was crawl into bed. Right now I feel like I have a massive
hangover and I'm struggling to concentrate on what I'm
writing. Hopefully I'll wake up tomorrow feeling refreshed and
clear in the head because we are off to Vegas!*

Yeah, sure, I've been saying that for two years!

14 September 2008

*It's time to 'vivre' Las Vegas. We have been here less than
one day and I can confidently say that if eating, drinking
and gambling is what you love to do, then this place is your
paradise. If not, and for me it most definitely isn't, then I think
forty-eight hours is more than enough. We are staying in the
fanciest hotel we have been in in the four months we have
been away. We visited a show last night and indulged in a
delicious dinner. I'd run 15km in the morning so I managed to
enjoy it.*

*Off to Boston tomorrow for 5 days, followed by LA, San
Francisco then Auckland to visit friends. Brent is flying back
home to start a new job tomorrow so it's time to fly solo*

again. Still feeling unbalanced and dizzy, the odd sensations in my legs are still there. I really think these demons are with me for life ...

1 October 2008

I am in Auckland visiting Paddy, a good friend from uni. After nearly four weeks hopping around the US I want to stay put. I'm sick of packing and unpacking my bags, sleeping in different beds and eating out every night.

I am so tired. And I am so sick of feeling like this. I thought five months away would cure me and I'd return home feeling normal, this horrible unknown illness all but a distant memory.

It has been the adventure of a lifetime and I have conquered challenges I never thought possible, but I just want to feel NORMAL. Let me enjoy walking down the street feeling in control of my body. Let me enjoy going for a run. Let me enjoy life.

Today I tried explaining to Paddy how I felt. He pretended to understand, but I know he thought I was insane and that upsets me so much. In two days I'll be home, back to reality, back to work and most likely, back to searching for an explanation to these horrible symptoms.

It's all too much to bear.

17

Lessons not learnt

10 October 2008

To be honest, it's not great to be back. It was wonderful seeing family and friends after so long away and unpacking my bags and sleeping in my own bed, but I'm over that now.

This is it, there's no more travelling, no more adventures, just the same routine every single day — at least for a while.

I am living in the same apartment in Port Melbourne but Brent has moved in. It's only temporary until we find a place of our own. I am doing casual teaching at Melbourne University in the Department of Physiotherapy but I don't think I will return to practising as a physio. Not until I feel completely well again.

I saw Trevor yesterday for the first time in five months. He told me I'm looking well — I wish I felt it. Now that my energy levels are one hundred per cent I think I'll just see him every few months for a 'tune up'.

By the end of October Brent and I had settled back into our life in Melbourne. I continued to exercise as much as possible every day — running in the morning, cycling to and from work and walking for an hour at lunchtime. I would then collapse on the couch at night, emotionally drained and utterly exhausted from trying to get through the day with my persistent symptoms.

I was still caught up in a constant battle, with the voice in my head reminding me that kilojoule output had to equal input or else I would end up a big fat slob. It was an irrational, delusional way of thinking that I knew was not doing anything to get my health back on track, but I felt powerless to do anything about it. I continued to ignore my mid-morning hunger pains and waited until lunchtime to eat my salad and apple. That would be it until dinner. I found myself surviving on fewer and fewer kilojoules and was well aware that it was detrimental to my health but didn't have the strength to overcome my obsession and live my life the way I advised others to do.

'What do you think about moving to Singapore?' Brent asked me less than one month after returning from our overseas trip. 'I've seen a couple of great jobs online. We could move there for a couple of years.'

My initial thought was, Yes, let's go! I felt trapped in the monotony of everyday life and was itching to start moving again. There was a problem. What would I do there? I am not the housewife type. Being a lady of leisure would be great for a while, but I was sure to be bored after a couple of months. I need challenges and mental stimulation, to finish each day knowing I have achieved something.

'Sounds great honey,' I replied. 'But what am I going to do over there?'

'Maybe you could teach at a university,' Brent replied as if he had already thought it through. 'They must have a physiotherapy course in Singapore.'

I went online and searched for physiotherapy courses in

Singapore. The search found one match. There was a place called Nanyang Polytechnic (NYP), which offered the Diploma of Physiotherapy. I explored their website and clicked on job vacancies. I certainly didn't expect that the first advertised position would be for a physiotherapy lecturer.

'Apply now,' Brent said when I told him.

Brent usually likes to think things through, but it sounded as if he already had his mind set on moving to Singapore.

'What are the chances of you being offered a job?' I asked. 'I don't want to apply if you're not serious about going.'

'If you're keen to move, then so am I. Why don't we both apply and see what happens?' he replied.

'Okay,' I said. 'Why not? I'm ready for another adventure.'

So I compiled my resume and applied for the position as physiotherapy lecturer at Nanyang Polytechnic. Brent applied for advertised positions as Director of Tennis at two expatriate clubs.

A week later I received a phone call from the Physiotherapy Manager and Director of the School of Health Sciences at Nanyang Polytechnic. After an informal one-hour phone interview, we arranged a time the following week for a formal interview via teleconference. I arranged to have the interview in a boardroom in the School of Medicine at TheUniversity of Melbourne and felt miniscule as I sat down to a table large enough to seat twenty people.

A panel of four filled the enormous screen that covered the wall at the far end of the room: two staff from the Human Resources department and the Director and Deputy Director of the School of Health Sciences. They greeted me as I entered their view. I knew Singaporeans were very particular in their processes and procedures, so I expected them to ask innumerable questions and quiz me on every aspect of my resume.

I wasn't surprised when I was informed that Singaporeans work harder and longer than Australians and they have stricter work policies and procedures. They asked if I would be able to adapt to this kind of working environment.

'Yes, of course,' I replied confidently. 'I have worked overseas before and love new challenges.' (I didn't explain that my previous work overseas was in a very casual working environment in Phuket as an English teacher.)

After over an hour of interrogation the interview came to a close and I was informed that I would be told the outcome in six weeks. I walked out of the conference room not quite sure what to think. I was quietly confident about my chances of being offered the position but adapting to their work ethics and environment was going to be more of a challenge than I had initially anticipated.

I couldn't believe I was standing at the start line of a race, up against hundreds of other runners. After more than two years out of serious training and racing, Brent had encouraged me to enter the ten-kilometre Sussan Women's Fun Run, an annual run held exclusively for women.

I had been completing the distance several times per week for over a year, so I knew I could finish the race, but I was concerned about how I would feel during the run as there were no signs of my symptoms diminishing. I was also up against a psychological challenge. It was going to be difficult to accept that I would not run anywhere near as fast as my personal best time of 38.30 minutes, and I would be beaten by women who would have been no competition for me previously.

I had to accept that I was not the runner I once was and that a year ago, I would have done anything just to run a race. I tried to convince myself that I would be happy with a time around fifty minutes. Anything faster would be a bonus.

I began the race a few rows back from the start line. Gone were the days when I politely forced my way to the front. I no longer belonged there. I glanced at the runners out in front, kitted out in their two-piece lycra gear, their abdominal muscles prominent. I used to be one of them, I thought. I used to have a defined stomach with six visible packs of muscle.

Although still lean, I didn't think I looked like a marathon runner any more and I tried to shut down the part of me wishing I looked like them. It's not healthy, I tried to convince myself. Looking back at photos from this race, I didn't look much different from the elite runners, but my warped mind saw me differently.

The race went well. The dizziness set in at about the five-kilometre mark but didn't worsen and the constricted feelings in my legs were constant but bearable. I ran the first half in just under twenty-two minutes and the second half nearly one minute faster. I was shocked but elated as I crossed the line in 43.08 minutes.

Brent cheered me on from the sidelines and as always, was there to see me cross the finish line. I crossed the line with my arms overhead, feeling as triumphant as I had felt at the end of the Melbourne Marathon. A year ago I could never have imagined I would ever be crossing a finish line again. I ran straight into Brent's arms, his firm, prolonged embrace enough to tell me just how proud he was. I never thought that a ten-kilometre fun run could turn out to be such an emotional and momentous occasion.

Four months after arriving home we were packing our bags once again, this time for Singapore. We left Melbourne with five suitcases, ten boxes and a bike: one hundred and twenty kilograms in total.

It's always exciting arriving in a new city, feeling like a total stranger in a foreign culture, meeting intriguing people, exploring unknown surroundings, peculiar smells and unfamiliar food. For the best part of a month Brent and I felt like we were on holiday, exploring and discovering the diversity that Singapore has to offer. We hunted for the best places to shop, we explored running and cycling routes and familiarised ourselves with the public transport system.

We were fortunate to be living on campus at the Polytechnic with access to a magnificent running track, a gym and a fifty-metre pool. Brent and I settled into our jobs, adapting well to the disparate working environment.

To say that I stood out amongst the staff at NYP is an understatement. Within a few weeks many people had met or heard of the new 'Ang Mo' (Chinese for foreigner) either walking around or running laps of the campus. I ran early in the morning to beat the heat. The humidity was immense and it made my first few runs a tremendous effort. Initially I struggled to run more than six kilometres but as I began to acclimatise, six kilometres became eight, which turned into ten. On days when I felt the need to burn extra energy, I would clock up to fourteen kilometres. My sweat glands worked overtime to dissipate the extreme heat and I could wring the sweat from my clothes after each run.

Outside of work there was not much else to do and Brent was often not home before ten at night so I found myself with extra time to exercise and obsess over how many kilojoules I had consumed. Despite my nagging symptoms, my energy levels were fine so in addition to running, I began swimming two days per week and going to the gym after work. Two swimming sessions quickly became three and before I knew it I was doing some form of exercise before work, at lunchtime and after work every day of the week. With a pool, running track and gym at my doorstep, I couldn't resist the temptation to burn more kilojoules.

My symptoms persisted but they were no different whether I exercised or not. My eating habits remained the same, limiting my intake during the day only to give in at night and indulge in cereal and yogurt. On so many occasions, as I had done for several years, I began an exercise session feeling hungry but I ignored it and the feeling soon passed. I had to earn my food first.

It had been a little over two months since we moved to Singapore when I returned home from work after a trying day, overwhelmed by the severity of my symptoms. I had already run ten kilometres that morning but I was so angry with my body that I felt the urge to punish and torture it for putting me through this neverending nightmare. So I did exactly that. I headed to the track and started running a few laps.

I struggled to stay within my lane but I ignored the unsteadiness, determined to give my body the beating it deserved. I ran faster. I pushed harder. Five laps, ten laps, twenty laps, thirty laps. Come on, I urged myself. Push harder. Make it hurt. Feel the pain. You deserve it. Forty laps. My eyes began to blur from the tears streaming down my face. I finally realised what I was doing and stopped, so dizzy I almost fell over. I was satisfied with the punishment.

As I was leaving the track a man approached me and introduced himself as Andrew. He was the running coach of the track team at the Polytechnic and Singapore's national middle-distance coach. He told me he was impressed with my running style and commented that I looked very fit. He asked what distances I ran and what my best times were. I proudly told him that I had run a sub-three-hour marathon – an achievement I can and will always claim. Being part of this elusive sub-three-hour club gains you automatic respect from fellow runners and Andrew asked me if I was keen to run races competitively. If so, he would be able to organise a small deal for me with Nike.

The thought of returning to competition excited me and having a sponsor again was a dream come true. There was no way I was going to pass up this fantastic opportunity so I gave Andrew my phone number. He said he would be in touch regarding upcoming races and some free Nike gear.

I so desperately wanted to regain my health and to enjoy running again. What I would do just to be able to get through a run feeling normal, balanced, strong, in control of my body – exactly what I had taken for granted for so many years. I knew it was in my control, but I was too embarrassed to expose the chaos, the jumbled mess that was going on in my own mind. I still struggled to understand how eating more and exercising less would make my symptoms go away, but if I could speak to my old self I would say, 'Stop training three times per day. Stop forcing your body to exercise when it's tired. Don't deprive your body of the fuel it needs. Eat when you're hungry.'

It was so simple. Yet so complicated.

After running a few races I realised that my times, albeit far slower than my best, placed me in the category of elite runners in

Singapore and in the top three of most races. Within a year I was offered sponsorship with PowerBar and given priority access to the front line of every race I entered. The following year I found myself on advertisements for HTWO-O, one of the largest sports drink companies in Singapore.

Seeing my image on life-sized posters in train stations and around sporting tracks and universities was surreal. With the current times I was clocking, I didn't feel as if I deserved the recognition but I accepted it with gratitude. I was lean and toned and with my commendable results and a few sponsors attached to my name, I began to train harder. I was winning cash and great prizes so I entered races nearly every weekend.

The battle continued with the uncompromising voice in my head. I punished my body on the track with four-hundred-metre interval sessions and once a week I forced my way up seventy flights of stairs, my legs burning and my heart rate close to its maximum. I knew my symptoms would prevent me from improving my times but at least I was pushing my body to extreme and burning lots of kilojoules in the process.

The more intense sessions exacerbated my symptoms and left me unable to concentrate for the rest of the day, but my accomplishments provided me with satisfaction. The interval sessions increased to three per week, then four times. My students told me they were amazed by my discipline and dedication and that I inspired them to exercise. I let them believe it, secretly ashamed that it was nothing short of an unhealthy obsession.

With this 'elite' status attached to my name, I felt an even greater pressure to maintain my runner's physique and continued to monitor my kilojoule intake, adamant not to consume more than what I expended through exercise, and disregarding the five thousand kilojoules per day I needed just to survive.

As clichéd as it sounds, from the moment I arrived in Phuket in November 2002, I knew Brent and I were meant to be together.

Set on a beautiful beach with a picturesque lagoon on one side, we both have a sentimental attachment to Laguna Beach Resort in Phuket. In August 2009, six months after our move to Singapore, we returned there for a holiday. We had enjoyed a delicious dinner at one of our favourite restaurants overlooking the ocean followed by a serene walk along the beach, the sound of the waves in the background. Brent broke out in a tune that he used to sing to me during our first year together and as it ended, he dropped to one knee, took my hands in his and asked the question I had been waiting to hear.

He reached into his pocket and pulled out a small box. He opened it to reveal a beautiful necklace with a small diamond embedded in a heart. Finally, I wanted to blurt out. But for once I thought before speaking and instead I yelled out, 'Yes!'

We hugged and kissed. I hadn't been this happy in a long time. Brent proposed with a necklace so I could choose my own engagement ring. I couldn't wait to go shopping. When we returned to our hotel room my jaw dropped at what lay before me. Our room was decorated with beautiful purple and white orchids and red roses. Two swans constructed using towels were propped up on the bed surrounded by rose petals that formed the word 'LOVE'. A bottle of champagne was waiting for us on the table. I looked at Brent in amazement.

'Did you organise this?' I asked before realising how stupid the question was.

I was so impressed and extremely touched by the effort and planning that had gone into making the night perfect. Neither of us really like champagne, but that night it tasted better than ever.

18

2010 Turning point

In March 2010, seven months after Brent proposed, we returned to Melbourne for our engagement party. We had decided to have a relatively small wedding in Thailand, at Laguna Beach Resort, so we wanted all our friends and family to help celebrate our engagement.

Before flying back to Melbourne I led a group of students to Cambodia on a Youth Expedition Project. We worked in orphanages and on a remote island off Phnom Penh building huts, providing clothes and stationery, teaching English and painting classrooms and bedrooms.

The expedition was extremely rewarding, but being responsible for twenty students and the conditions we endured – sharing a small house with no air-conditioning or running water, with the temperatures soaring into the mid thirties every day – made for a challenging two weeks. By the time I flew to Melbourne to join Brent, who had flown in a few days earlier, I was exhausted.

With three days until our engagement party, there was no time to rest. We helped Mum and Dad prepare nibbles for over one hundred and fifty people and set their house up for what was a fabulous afternoon – great company, humorous speeches and scrumptious food. I felt dizzy the entire day, but somehow managed to enjoy myself.

We set the big day for the beginning of August the same year. The few months leading up to the wedding were busy. In addition to my usual teaching load, I organised a second trip to Cambodia for students and a study trip to Melbourne – all while planning a wedding.

I lost count of the number of emails we exchanged with our wedding organiser in Thailand. The ceremony needed to be arranged, the flower arrangements, the songs and the celebrant. A hairdresser, photographer and videographer needed to be booked. For the reception, the table arrangements, food, flowers, decorations, music, lighting and cake all needed organising, too. I arranged accommodation for friends and family who were flying in from Australia, France, USA, Zimbabwe and Singapore and we went to Bangkok three months before the wedding to legalise our marriage. It was a lot of work, but I loved every minute.

The wedding was another incentive to stay thin and during the months leading up to it the voice became louder than ever. Despite my busy schedule I continued to train two to three times a day and averaged three races per month. I continued to do well in the races despite my persistent symptoms. I even squeezed in a race the day before departing for Thailand. The effort put into planning our wedding was worth it. It turned out to be a perfect day. A magical wedding overlooking a lagoon just metres from the beach with sixty close friends and family. It was a day we will both remember forever.

I have always wanted to have children and I don't know anyone who has wanted to become a father more than Brent. I had been taking the birth control pill for ten years except for a six-month break in 2006, when I realised that my reproductive system had shut down – another warning sign I chose to ignore.

A few weeks after our wedding Brent mentioned that I looked

smaller. It was his way of subtly telling me I needed to put on weight. He had told me many times before but my usual abrupt response made it clear that there was no point trying to reason with me and the conversation never evolved further.

'Have you lost more weight?' he asked.

'No,' I said. 'Why?'

'You just look thinner. Look at your arms. They're like twigs.'

'They are not,' I replied defensively. 'I'm fine. I'm winning races so I'm obviously at my perfect weight.'

This time Brent was more persistent.

'If we wanted to have kids now, would you be able to?' he asked.

I hadn't expected this question and it struck me like a bullet. I was speechless. What was I meant to say? Was I meant to lie to give him peace of mind? Or was I supposed to tell him the truth: that my reproductive system was currently dormant and I didn't know if I would be able to have children. Ever.

A feeling of guilt swept across my body as I shook my head, realising that I could no longer deny the fact that my unhealthy obsession was not only jeopardising my health, but our chances of starting a family. We were married, I was thirty, and whether I liked it or not, my biological clock was ticking.

We agreed that I should go off the pill again, this time with the aim of trying to fall pregnant. I didn't tell Brent that there was no way I would be ovulating. I decided to give it three months and see if my menstrual cycle resumed before considering fertility treatment. It was no surprise to me when it didn't. There wasn't even a hint that my reproductive system was functioning normally.

Every month Brent asked if there was any progress. I didn't want to expose my greatest fear to him: that I may have done permanent damage and I might never be able to fall pregnant. So each time my reply was the same. 'No, but it often takes a while when you come off the pill.'

Three months after I stopped taking the pill, with no signs of my period reappearing, I made an appointment with a fertility specialist to examine whether my reproductive system was anywhere near waking up. She made no comment on my weight but a couple of ultrasounds revealed the follicles were not growing, an indication that I was not even close to ovulating. I was told that my uterine lining was so thin that even if I did fall pregnant, I would most likely miscarry. As I had only been off the pill for a few months, the specialist wanted me to wait another couple of months to see if my body could do anything on its own before starting fertility treatment. I left the clinic feeling at an all-time low; disheartened, ashamed and guilty and wondering if I had done permanent damage to my reproductive system and destroyed any chance of starting a family, one of Brent's greatest desires.

As I had done a few years earlier, I spent hours on the internet searching for information. I wanted to find people with similar stories who had overcome adversity and fallen pregnant. I needed to be reassured that I hadn't irreversibly damaged my reproductive system.

I searched on athletic amenorrhoea and discovered a wealth of information. Some of what I read was encouraging, some was disheartening, but all the articles agreed on one thing: athletic amenorrhoea is caused by the stress of excessive exercise and insufficient kilojoule consumption resulting in low body fat. With extremely low body fat, the ovaries stop producing oestrogen, which is important for ovulation and protecting our bones. This explains why there is almost a three times higher incidence of stress fractures in athletes with amenorrhoea compared to those menstruating.

I had studied nutrition at university and this was all familiar information, but I had to read it over and over to accept how accurately it described me. I needed to see it written on the page in front of me. If I were to extract one dominant and consistent message from what I was reading it would be that amenorrhoea is a warning sign that the body is under too much stress and has too little energy stores to support healthy functioning. Something I had known all along but which I had chosen to discount.

As quickly as you can flick a switch, something transformed in my mind. Instantly, I was prepared to listen. I was willing to admit my mistakes and ultimately face them. I spent hours researching the management of athletic amenorrhoea but every article relayed the same message: reduce exercise and increase kilojoule consumption. To my disordered mind, I read this as: Sit on the couch and become a fat slob. It couldn't have been simpler, but I knew this was going to be the biggest challenge of my life.

It was encouraging to read the condition was reversible, but there was no knowing how long it would take to regain normal cycles. Some articles said six to twelve months. Twelve months? I thought in horror. Twelve months of eating more, exercising a lot less and putting on weight. It was a daunting prospect and I knew that I would have to fight and conquer the voice in my head.

The most frightening part was that there was no guarantee I would fall pregnant. Twelve months down the track I could be fat, unfit and not pregnant. And still ridden with horrible symptoms. There was no magic number of kilograms I had to put on for my menstrual cycle to return. It could be five, ten, even fifteen kilograms. I dreaded putting on weight. People are going to think I'm pregnant when I'm not, I thought.

I didn't want to discuss my fear with Brent because I was embarrassed and I didn't think he would understand just how difficult it was going to be. I spent hours on the internet searching for alternate solutions. But there were none.

During my search I came across a forum called Fertile Thoughts, a discussion board for people with hypothalamic amenorrhoea – a name for amenorrhoea caused by depression of the hypothalamus. This is most commonly due to negative energy balance (more kilojoules expended than consumed), resulting in very low body fat.

This forum became the turning point for me. Most of the women on the board had a history of eating disorders and exercise addiction. I was encouraged by those with similar stories to mine who had wondered if they would ever fall pregnant and who, after making the necessary lifestyle changes, had eventually had children.

For some it had taken a few months, others two or three years. Many had spent thousands of dollars on unsuccessful fertility treatments, only to fall pregnant naturally after reducing their exercise and putting on weight: after listening to their body and giving it the love and care it deserved.

While reading the blogs a light bulb suddenly switched on in my head and everything became so clear. As I read other people's accounts of their exercise addiction and eating patterns, I couldn't help thinking how detrimental their lifestyle must be to their health. How could they live like this and not get sick? I wondered. How can they keep punishing their bodies day after day? How can they live on so few kilojoules?

Some had posted photos of themselves. Most looked unhealthy, some emaciated, their shoulders protruding and their faces gaunt. The health professional in me wanted to write to them and tell them to put on weight. To stop exercising and to start eating. I realised that what I wanted to say to these people was what others had been telling me for years.

Suddenly my perception of myself and my life changed. I looked in the mirror and the woman looking back was the person who, for many years, had been told to slow down. To put on weight. To stop punishing her body. I could finally view her from the same perspective as others around me.

At last it dawned on me that I had spent over four years and thousands of dollars trying to find a cure for my physical symptoms, when I should have been seeking counselling to battle the voice in my head that had led me down the path of self-destruction. My lifestyle and my symptoms were nothing but a reflection of my sick, delusional mind.

I knew I had two options if I wanted to get pregnant. I wrote them both on a piece of paper so I could see them clearly.

1. *To continue to deny my obsession with exercise and my weight and spend thousands of dollars on fertility treatment, trying to convince myself that I can get pregnant without changing my lifestyle.*
2. *To stop exercising excessively and restricting kilojoules and to put on weight.*

It was indubitable which option to take.

Conquering the voice in my head and changing my distorted way of thinking to accept that I needed to put on weight and stop pushing my body so hard proved to be the biggest challenge in my journey to recovery, but it was the key to regaining my health.

I have always strived to reach my goals and when I have my mind set on something, I'll do whatever it takes to make it happen. My goal of getting pregnant was no exception. I knew the battle with the voice in my head would not be easily won and I would need visual reminders to conquer this psychological challenge. I found a piece of butcher's paper and in large black print wrote out my goals and how I planned to achieve them. I posted it to my bedroom wall.

1 December 2010
Ultimate goals:
- *Get pregnant*
- *Vanquish all symptoms*
- *Feel healthy*

Short-term goal:
Put on six kilograms by end of February 2011

How I am going to do it:
- *Exercise NO MORE than four times a week for NO MORE than thirty minutes at a time*
- *Eat carbohydrates with EVERY meal – breakfast, lunch and dinner*
- *Snack mornings and afternoons*
- *Consume more fats every day*
- *IGNORE the voice in my head – it is irrational, senseless and it is DESTROYING me.*

The day I set my goals I decided to join the Fertile Thoughts forum. My initial resistance to joining the forum was my denial in admitting I had a problem. I was embarrassed that my state of health and sedated reproductive system were not bad luck, but were self-inflicted. I was ashamed. And it was not only me who had suffered over the past few years, I had dragged my parents and Brent down with me. But after coming to terms with reality and reading stories from women who had shared their own journey, I decided to share mine. I found it easier disclosing my problem to strangers, and my first confession was instrumental in my recovery.

1 December 2010

Hi everyone,

I have been reading your blogs for a couple of months. I am so grateful to learn so much from you and to know that there are other people out there in a similar situation to me and most importantly, who think the same way I do – that I HAVE to exercise every day.

I am 31 years old, previously an elite marathon runner, training up to a hundred and fifty kilometres a week. That was a few years ago. In 2006 I became very sick. Extreme fatigue, dizziness and brain fog are just a few of the horrible symptoms I suffered and continue to endure. I have had hundreds of tests but nothing has been diagnosed.

The past two or three years my energy has been a hundred per cent, but I'm not able to run long distances any more. The symptoms are too bad and my body just won't let me, so I just run ten to twelve kilometres at a time. I compete in ten to fifteen kilometre races two to three times a month. I also cycle and swim.

I know I still exercise excessively (two to three times per day, seven days per week) but I can't help it and I love *knowing I am burning so much energy. For the past few years I couldn't have imagined doing any less and having a day off was out of the question.*

I have also restricted my diet for the past few years. I feel guilty when I consume more kilojoules than I burn through exercise. I have been very lean for a few years and I love it.

I went off the birth control pill three months ago after ten years and surprise, surprise, no period. My body fat is now twelve per cent and body mass index (BMI) is eighteen. Too low, I know.

A couple of recent ultrasounds revealed my follicles are not growing and my uterine lining is so thin that even if I did fall pregnant, I would most likely miscarry. After reading everyone else's stories on this forum, I have decided that as of today I am going to put on weight by reducing my exercise and eating more. I know it's not going to be easy, but I am determined to achieve my goal.

I look forward to getting to know you all and sharing my journey with you.

As with all challenges in my life, I approached this one with determination. Failing to achieve my goals was not an option. Forget 'gradually' reducing my exercise. I didn't want this to take months – I wanted it now. Overnight I went from exercising two to three hours a day, seven days a week to thirty minutes a day, four days a week.

Increasing my kilojoule intake wasn't quite as easy so I introduced carbohydrates and fats more gradually. I began by eating a piece of a toast with fruit and yogurt at breakfast. A week later I replaced my salad at lunch with a sandwich and the following week the vegetables that had previously filled my dinner plate made way for some pasta or rice. Within three weeks, carbohydrates, which I previously consumed only on special occasions, filled half my plate at every meal. I ate snacks every two hours, some healthy, others not so healthy, and before long, Nutella and peanut butter sandwiches were a staple part of my diet.

The voice that had controlled me for so long did not dissipate completely into thin air however. I was still keeping track of the number of kilojoules that entered my body but I was given some leeway, a margin of safety which allowed me to consume a lot more than I had for years without being ridden with guilt.

Over the next two months I spent every night on the forum, reading other women's posts and giving an update on my progress. It was similar to keeping a diary, only this time I received responses. It was great to be in touch with women who really understood where I was coming from and just how difficult it was to reduce my exercise and put on weight. I was so grateful for their invaluable advice and endless support. Reading stories from women on the board who had turned their lives around and fallen pregnant provided reassurance and helped me remain focused on my goals. To my surprise, I didn't balloon out like a whale within a week as had been my fear for so many years. This proved how deprived my body had been for so long. The extra kilojoules did not go straight to my hips, instead they helped my body recuperate and function at full capacity.

I was determined to do anything to achieve my goal and after reading articles suggesting that cold foods reduce fertility, I eliminated ice cream and salads from my diet. I started acupuncture and consumed Chinese herbs after reading about their fertility benefits. I was doing everything to enhance my chances of conceiving and at the same time, to improve my health.

I woke up one morning in early January and headed to the gym. It was one of my allowed days of exercise. I started working out on the cross-trainer and before I knew it, the timer reached thirty minutes. Time was up. I felt an enormous temptation to go just another five minutes. What difference will five minutes make? I thought. I kept going. Thirty-one minutes. Thirty-two minutes. Maybe I can go for an hour today. Just today. The voice in the background urged me to continue. You'll be allowed extra food if you go for longer. Burn more and you can eat more.

Only a couple of months earlier I would have given in. I would have obeyed the voice, convinced that another five minutes could only do me good. I would have pushed harder, filling my legs with lactic acid in an effort to burn as much energy as possible.

I pictured the thick, black writing on the butcher's paper posted on my bedroom wall. There was no-one else in the gym so I yelled my goals out: 'Get pregnant, vanquish all symptoms, feel healthy!' I stopped and stepped off the cross-trainer. It was one small victory.

My willpower was tested again a week later when I was due to compete in a triathlon that I had entered three months earlier. There was generous prize money for the first three place-getters and I knew I had a good chance of winning. It had been six weeks since I set my goals and I found myself torn between whether I should race or not. Surely one race won't hurt, one part of me said. What difference will it make? Another part of me knew it would be stupid to compete. What is more important, winning cash or regaining your health and having a baby?

I decided to get confirmation from my friends on the board. I explained my situation and asked for their advice. I received many replies, all advising against competing. One reply left the greatest impression: 'Baby or trophy?' My decision was made.

For the next month I continued to refrain from running every morning. When I did run, it was for no more than thirty minutes and at a low intensity. I had a lot of spare time when I would usually have been pounding the pavement, hitting the gym or swimming laps. I needed to find another hobby, to focus my mind elsewhere and distract me from the fact that I could be exercising and burning kilojoules.

I decided to write a book. I wanted, one day, when I was completely healthy and blessed with a beautiful child, to share my story with others. I wanted to warn others of how a healthy hobby can so quickly become a dangerous obsession. By demonstrating the depths of my obsession and the miracle of my recovery, I wanted to prevent others falling into the same trap. I wanted to show people who are in a similar situation that there is a way forward.

Although I still had to draw on an enormous amount of mental strength and willpower, over time it became easier to wake up and eat breakfast without exercising first. There were times when I felt as if a powerful force was trying to suck me back into my old lifestyle, but I reminded myself of why I was doing this.

I was surprised how long it took to put on weight considering the amount I was eating and how little I was exercising. During the first two months I put on four kilograms. My body fat increased to twenty per cent and my BMI to twenty-one.

Not being able to squeeze into my skinny jeans and feeling every small roll on my stomach, which had previously felt as hard as an ironing board, was not a pleasant feeling. I continued to ask myself the questions, Where did I want to be in one year's time? Did I want to be lean, still suffering horrible symptoms and trying to fall pregnant? Or did I want to be healthy and pregnant? Or better still, holding a baby?

When Brent and I moved back to Melbourne from Singapore at the beginning of March 2011, I was six kilograms heavier than I had been three months earlier. When I saw people who I hadn't seen since our wedding, I almost heard their inner voices saying, Gee, she's put on weight. But I realise now that it was just my irrational mind speaking, and friends have since told me that when they first saw me after we moved back to Melbourne their initial thought was how much healthier I looked.

There continued to be days when the voice almost prevailed and I felt an overpowering urge to push my body that little bit harder or to exercise for sixty minutes instead of thirty minutes. There were moments of guilt for finishing a bowl of pasta or the chunky potato chips that covered half my dinner plate. I couldn't believe how much bread I was eating or how many desserts I was devouring.

More of my clothes began to feel tight and I struggled to fit into my running clothes, but I reminded myself of my ultimate goals and continued on my journey to recovery. I started to enjoy the lifestyle my body had been craving for so long. I was beginning to feel healthier and because I could enjoy delicacies without guilt, I looked forward to social events more than I had done in six years.

By the middle of March I had put on seven kilograms and my symptoms had subsided dramatically. Two weeks later I discovered I was pregnant.

Epilogue

As I sit here with my beautiful daughter in my arms, I can't stop thinking how fortunate I am.

I fell pregnant at the end of March 2011, almost four months after making the promise to myself to reduce my exercise and put on weight. During that time I put on seven kilograms and increased my body fat from twelve to twenty-two per cent.

Having fallen pregnant so quickly, I consider myself one of the lucky ones. I know that many women on the forum are still battling their inner demons and trying to start a family. I met one of the women, Anna, in person just after I fell pregnant. We have been great friends since and now my daughter has a friend to play with as Anna reached her ultimate goal eight months after making a similar promise to herself.

I continued to limit my exercise schedule while I was pregnant, running only a few times per week, and no more than thirty minutes at a time. I fuelled my body as it desired. My symptoms began to subside just before I fell pregnant and had disappeared completely one month before I gave birth – more than five years after I embarked on what I hope was the most devastating and distressing journey I will ever have to endure. It was horrific and unnerving not only for myself, but for my loved ones too.

Despite the anguish and suffering I and the people close to me endured and the depths of despair I found myself drowning in, I consider the journey I have been on over the past six years a blessing. It was by far the most challenging time of my life – and there were moments when I felt like giving up – but I know it was the only way to force me to stop torturing myself and pushing my body so hard.

When people ask me what caused me to punish myself with such an extreme lifestyle, I don't have an answer, but the word control comes to mind. Sometimes the choices we make in life reflect our history and upbringing and create our destiny, but sometimes things just happen. I believe I fit the latter. I thrived on the control I had over my body, on testing the boundaries and pushing it to its absolute limit. I am strong-minded, strong-willed and will do whatever it takes to achieve goals I set out for. In this case, I paid a hefty price. When I reflect on my journey, I am surprised at my lack of introspection. That even my firsthand experience with children whose lives are a constant struggle, who were neglected and left to die on doorsteps by their parents wasn't enough to take my focus off my running and make me realise the important things in life. It wasn't enough to make me realise that being fast, lean and athletic is not the most important thing in the world. But as I have told my story, it is only now I understand the web of confusion I had become entangled in and how blinded I was by my obsession. In denial and unaware of the damage I was doing to myself, this self-sabotaging young woman feels distant to me now. She is nothing but a stranger for whom I feel a great amount of sympathy.

I naively and stubbornly brushed off advice from medical experts to reduce my training load and put on weight and I refused to listen to family and friends. To me they were ignorant, their advice far from credible. I completed every training session at the highest intensity possible and in absolute denial of the damage I was doing to my body. Ignoring the initial physical warning

signs – stress fractures and absent menstruation – and refusing to
believe that they were a result of my actions, I pushed on. I was in a
constant battle with my body which continued to cry out for help.
Eventually it took drastic measures, and I was reduced to absolute
exhaustion as it inflicted on me a seemingly never-ending list of
disturbing symptoms.

The human body is a weird and wonderful thing and although
there is still is a lot to be discovered about it, we do know that the
body needs food to survive – and it is not designed to endure the
gruelling training I subjected mine to. Now that I am detached
from the person I once was, looking in from the outside, I see all
too clearly what everyone around me could see all along. And I am
proud to say that the self-absorbed woman who left Brent perched
on the edge of a mountain over four thousand metres above sea
level, breathless and hallucinating, in order to conquer the physical
challenge set before her and reach her goal, the selfish, troubled
person whose life revolved around running and being lean is a
stranger to me now.

My desire to have a baby was the turning point in my journey.
When Brent and I started talking about having children, I was
struck with an enormous sense of guilt that I may not be able to
fall pregnant and I knew I had to change the way I was living my
life – fast. I knew this was going to be my biggest challenge yet – a
battle I had to fight with myself and with the voice. I also knew
that as with all challenges set before me, losing was not an option.
My pregnancy however wasn't a miraculous cure and my recovery
didn't happen overnight. There were times during my pregnancy
when I still felt dizzy and unbalanced and thought it would never
end. I wondered how I would be able to look after a baby feeling

so unwell. But from the moment I made a promise to my body to look after myself and vowed never to return to my former lifestyle, I gradually began to feel well again.

I believe my illness was my body's way of saying enough is enough. It felt threatened by my infinite discipline and determination to push it to its limit and the symptoms were its way of rebelling. It is no coincidence that I started feeling well when my mindset changed and I started looking after myself.

After one year of limiting my exercise and not worrying about what I put in my mouth, my body re-established its trust in me. I have no doubt that had I not had the desire to start a family, I would still be battling the voice in my head and suffering horrible symptoms, blindly searching for a cure, and for someone else who could fix me. I would never have had to confess to and face my mistakes.

Although it seemed like the end of the world when my competitive running days were forced to an end and I will always regret not reaching my full potential as a runner, my journey has helped me to appreciate and be thankful for everything in my life. I realise now how much I used to take for granted: my family, my friends and my health. There will always be a sense of regret when I reflect on this time in my life but I am a better person because of what I experienced. A better mother and a better friend.

I am ever so grateful to my friends who have stuck by me over the years despite the fact that I neglected them when training was my priority and then during the depths of my illness. I am very fortunate to have them all in my life.

I also feel absolutely blessed to have met Trevor, the kinesiologist who not only restored my energy levels but who provided ongoing support each and every time I visited him. I always left his clinic feeling more positive than when I arrived. I have referred many people to him for various health ailments and I go to see him occasionally when my body feels a little run down and in need of a little 'tune up'.

I would not have made it to the other end without the support of my loved ones, who not once pointed the finger at me and said, 'I told you so.' My parents are the most admirable people I know and I cannot thank them enough for their unconditional love and support during this journey, as always. They never gave up on me, even when I felt like giving up on myself. I am truly sorry for all the heartache and pain they were forced to endure.

Most of all, I am so lucky that my husband stuck by me during this rollercoaster ride. He is unfailing in his support and dedication, and to this day, considering how self-centred and unfair I was, I can't believe he stood by me during my illness. But I am ever so grateful he did and sorry for what he endured. I know my exercise addiction put immense strain on our relationship and I truly regret the months we had apart. He continues to support me in everything I set out to do and is the best husband and father anyone could ask for.

And finally, the exhilaration and excitement I felt from running marathons and pushing my body to the limit does not even come close to the immense happiness and elation that my beautiful daughter rewards me with every day. Occasionally I glance at my racing shoes – the shoes that took me to a sub-three-hour marathon time – and I wish I could be that good again, run that fast, effortlessly and fluently for endless kilometres. I thrived on pushing my body hard, cautious but unaware of its limits, and there are still times when I miss that feeling. Very rarely, I look at my size extra small crop top and lycra running shorts that I wore during the Melbourne Marathon and wonder what it would feel like to fit into them again. But very quickly I am brought back to reality, to what's important, by my little bundle of joy; her facial expressions, boundless affection and heart-warming smiles are priceless.

I began running again two weeks after giving birth, but these days I run for fun and to keep fit. I don't go to the extreme. I no longer feel compelled to run for two hours but am satisfied with a thirty-minute jog. I am currently completing a Doctor of Philosophy in Indigenous health, I lecture in sports medicine and I teach Pilates four times a week, which is great for increasing my core strength, and it provides a balance to my exercise routine and working life. Life is extremely busy and sometimes challenging but I wouldn't have it any other way.

I continue to follow a healthy diet and on very rare occasions my internal calculator can't help but estimate how many kilojoules I have consumed, but I say yes to desserts (sometimes even two) and I don't beat myself up about it afterwards. Rather, I enjoy them. I look forward to social gatherings and I enjoy the delicacies that come with them.

I have hips now – women are supposed to – and my body is no longer deprived of the energy and nutrients it needs. I lost most of my pregnancy weight within twelve months of having my daughter and have no desire to return to what I used to consider my 'ideal running weight'. I have maintained the same healthy weight the past year and had no trouble conceiving for a second time. Brent and I are very excited about the new addition to our family, due in less than three months.

Will I ever run another marathon? Deep down I would love to, but I know for now that my body doesn't want to and I am okay with that. Whether or not I do run another marathon, from now on I will be a lot smarter. I will listen to my body, I will give it rest when it wants it and I will fuel it properly.

To anyone who is training intensely or restricting kilojoules (or maybe doing both), living each and every day with the aim of being as lean as possible, I would ask you to consider what you are doing to your body. There is no doubt that you are extremely fit if you are running or hitting the gym every day, but are you healthy? And consider the facts below, in your own time and in your own way. I am sure to most people they are nothing new – indeed I knew them all along – but for so long I chose to ignore them.

1. *Women are not born to be marathon runners.*
2. *Women are supposed to have body fat, especially to bear children.*
3. *Running is not the most important thing in the world – there is much more to life.*
4. *Men like women with curves (well, most do anyway).*
5. *Being leaner doesn't make you happier.*
6. *The mind is a powerful thing. It can heal the body but you have to believe it will happen and provide it with the optimal environment.*
7. *Western medicine does not have an answer for everything. Sometimes you feel unwell, not because you are unwell, but simply because your body is crying out for some tender loving care.*
8. *Your body knows best. If you listen to it, love it and cherish it, it will do what you want it to. If you do not, it will send out signals to you in every way, shape and form.*
9. *Family and friends are more important than anything else.*

*Cherish them. The truly good ones will stick by you through the
difficult times.*
10. I am not invincible as my naive self once thought I was. No-one is.

As a last thought, two recent experiences have reinforced how
far I have come and how my priorities have changed. The first
incident was at a takeaway restaurant where Brent and I were
ordering pizza. Two young men and a young, slender woman
walked in. One of the men asked the woman what she wanted.

'Nothing,' she replied. 'I'm not hungry.'

'I haven't seen you eat all weekend,' he said as he shook his head.
'You need to eat. It's not healthy.'

I looked at the girl who was staring at the ground, obviously
embarrassed but unsure how to react. I knew she was hungry and
she wanted to eat pizza, but she was being controlled by a powerful
voice inside her head telling her she would get fat and would be
ridden with guilt if she did.

I desperately wanted to tell her that I understood what she was
thinking. I wanted to tell her to fight that voice and that being
healthy, enjoying all foods and nourishing your body is so much
more important than being thin. I wanted to share my journey, but
didn't know her, so I didn't say anything. I hope she and women
like her read my story.

The second incident was at a fitness expo I attended for work.
Women were walking around in skimpy gym gear showing off their
chiselled athletic physiques. As I walked around with my husband
and baby, I didn't feel a hint of jealousy towards them. Actually,
I felt sympathy because their lives were controlled by their strict
training routine, leaving little time for much else. I empathised

with them for having to follow a strict diet and denying themselves scrumptious foods.

I don't care that I no longer have a six-pack to show off. Nor do I care that I will probably never fit into my cute, extra small crop tops and bike pants again. What I care about is that I continue to feel well, I have the energy to be a good mother and wife, I enjoy running without racing against the clock and that I remain healthy.

Fit *and* healthy.

Acknowledgements

I've been blessed with a fabulous agent in Lyn Tranter who believed in me and my work from the beginning. Thank you so much for giving me a chance and for your ongoing support. I am extremely grateful to the team at Finch Publishing, especially Samantha Miles, Rex Finch and Laura Boon who have been so approachable and wonderful to work with and from whom I have learnt so much. I thank you from the bottom of my heart for all your support and guidance.

I give my heartfelt thanks to Kasey Edwards, an inspirational, intelligent author who passed on her knowledge and gave me the confidence to go ahead and publish my story. To Robina Smith, thank you for your invaluable advice. To Anna Vassallo, who has become such a great friend, thanks so much for your encouragement and for always being there to listen.

I feel extremely fortunate to have met Trevor Checuti, whose expertise and compassion goes beyond the call of duty and who listened tirelessly and remained optimistic for so long. Thank you for your care and support and for never giving up on me.

To my friends who have been with me along the way – you know who you are – and who have not judged me, I cannot thank you enough.

It is not merely enough to acknowledge the love and support from my family – my parents and my brother, Steve – no words can fully express my appreciation and love towards them. Without them, I wouldn't be where I am now and this book would not have been possible. To my mum and dad, my roles models in every aspect of life, the most admirable people I know, I will forever be grateful for your unquestioning support and unconditional love. Thank you for always believing in me, for encouraging me to follow my dreams and for never giving up on me. Thanks also for the endless cooked meals, babysitting duties and just for always being there.

To my wonderful husband Brent, my best friend, my other half. Words cannot express how grateful I am for your unwavering love, support and endless patience, not only throughout my journey, but during the endless days and nights I spent writing and editing this book. You stuck by me through the most challenging times and I would not have got through it without you . Your stamina and proficiency as a father made this book possible. Thank you so much for everything you do for your girls.

And finally to my beautiful daughters Mia and Madison, who made me realise what is important in life. Not only do you bring me balance in life, but the exhilaration I felt from running marathons does not even compare to the immense happiness and elation that you reward me with every day.